Ruth Ostrow has been a writer and journalist for over fifteen years. During the turbulent '80s and whilst working for the *Financial Review* newspaper she interviewed our top business leaders for her book, *The New Boy Network* which revealed the psychology and secrets of success of powerful men, and which became a national bestseller.

After a stint as the Tel Aviv editor of *Israel Economist*, Ruth moved to New York where she witnessed profound changes to the male-dominated corporate culture, which ultimately led her into writing about the men's movement, and finally about the impact the gender revolution was having on male–female relationships.

On her return from Manhattan Ruth became a social commentator, columnist and satirist for *The Australian* newspaper, combining her quirky sense of humour with her years of journalistic experience, before she joined the News Limited Sunday papers where she now has her own national, weekly page writing about sexuality and relationships.

hot &
sweaty

Ruth Ostrow

PAN
Pan Macmillan Australia

First published 1997 in Pan by Pan Macmillan Australia Pty Limited
St Martins Tower, 31 Market Street, Sydney

Acknowledgement: Several of the pieces in this book
have previously appeared in News Limited publications.

National Library of Australia
cataloguing-in-publication data:

Ostrow, Ruth, 1960–
Hot & sweaty.

ISBN 0 330 35982 7.

1. Interpersonal relations — Humor. 2. Love — Humor. 3.
Sex — Humor. I. Title.

A828.302

Typeset in 12/14pt Bembo by Post Typesetters
Printed in Australia by Australian Print Group

To my husband Morris, my soul-mate and liberator

ACKNOWLEDGMENTS

I would like to thank my:
Editors-in-chief at News Limited for their continued belief in me; Sunday editors who have allowed me room to explore; friends and family for their endless love and support; my agent David; assistant Christy; the warm staff at Pan Macmillan; and especially my readers who, through their letters, have taught me so much.

PREFACE

Each week my mailbox is like a confessional booth, full of words from hot and sweaty people who want to express themselves. Reading the first lines of some of the letters I have received over the years and which are peppered throughout this book, gives some idea of what I lay witness to.

'Dear Ruth, I would like to know why is pornography such a bad thing when it helps me learn about sex and how to enjoy it to the fullest? I am a twenty-nine-year-old mother of three'; 'Dear Ruth, I am a twenty-eight-year-old woman and partake in self-pleasure quite regularly and absolutely love it'; 'Dear Ruth, I use prostitutes on a regular basis.'

'Dear Ruth, I am a so-called "screamer" whilst making love'; 'Dear Ruth, I am a man in my late twenties with strong desires to indulge in anal penetration'; 'Dear Ruth, I am a man with a very small penis and I feel embarrassed'; 'Dear Ruth, what a relief to actually read in a mainstream newspaper that I am not so strange after all. I have enjoyed rubber clothing for as long as I can remember.'

A whispered admission from a lone soul in some anonymous street rising up to join the other whispered admissions from other lone souls, until there is a murmur and then a loud hum and then suddenly there are hundreds and hundreds of brave voices screaming out of my mailbox each week creating a dynamic and invigorating cacophony of sound. The sound of the truth.

These brilliant, funny, poignant and challenging letters tell it like it is, and they have always given me courage and insight, moved me to tears of laughter and sadness, but mainly they have inspired me to write this book.

For *Hot & Sweaty* is essentially my giant letter back to the world. A letter about liberation and celebration of our sexual, emotional and spiritual selves – which are all one and the same. It is a letter which answers my readers' need for acceptance, tolerance and love. Because if there is one message at the heart of my writing it is this: Come out!

Come out of the closet of your mind, and be free. Come out of the closet of other people's expectations, limitations, judgments, and dare to be happy. Come out and celebrate yourself for what you are: kinky, straight, bent, happily-married, male, female, dominant, submissive, monogamous, homosexual, bisexual or just sexual.

We are, none of us, long for this world.

Come out and play.

Contents

CHAPTER ONE

HOT BABES:

A road map
to women in the '90s

IT is a hot, smouldering night in New York City. The temperature inside one of New York's steamiest clubs is soaring up the
thermometer as bodies rub too close under the grind of funk
music. Suddenly the stage lights up. A host of women burst out.
They are dressed in the most erotic, tantalising garments imag-
inable.

Flimsy lace hardly covers the voluptuous body of one black
woman, another girl is in nothing but a G-string. The music
starts and the women move to various poles on the stage and
start performing in a way that is making the audience giddy.
Dainty, frilly things and sexy leather things are being thrown
into the gasping audience as graphic pornographic images
flicker on walls all over the room.

A woman dressed like a man with the appropriate plastic
attachment is gesturing lewdly in time to the music as the audience screams in delight. This could be any strip-club. But there
is something quite extraordinary going on here: the wild cheers

from the audience are not coming from men. Of the 500 or so patrons crammed into the huge, multi-level warehouse, there is not a man in sight.

This is one of New York's all-girl clubs. One of the new clubs run by women for women opening up all over the world. I have come here because I have heard about the sexplosion for women and I am curious about what is going on.

Some of the women here are gay, some are bi, but a fair few of the women I talk to over the course of the evening are straight – some married, others with kids – just out to have a fabulous evening unlocking the sexual energy that churns inside them.

It is a club where women proudly parade their fetishes and sexual bents, where women grab other women, and dance till dawn in a frenzy of sensuality and eroticism. It is a celebration of the sexual power of being female and it spits in the face of everything the so-called 'feminist thought police' tried to achieve in the '80s with their cry to political correctness.

'In here we can be totally free with our sexuality,' one twenty-three-year-old woman from London in latex and leather yells to me over the booming music. Her breasts are almost bare. 'I don't want to go to a club alone and be groped by men or leered at. But I want to go out and feel really turned on and sexy,' she yells before bumping off into the gyrating throng.

She is not alone in her views. The club is filled with lipstick feminists, goddess feminists, and sexy girls from the highest echelons of corporate America who, in step with the mother of erotic sleaze, Madonna, are following the call to 'express yourself'.

The outrageous success of clubs like this and like Europe's Pussy Posse which travels around Europe attracting hundreds of

women in every city, preaching fun, eroticism and safe sex –
teaching women to put condoms on with their mouths before
they go home – testifies to one fact. It is a fact backed up by the
burgeoning success of female sex-shops all over the world, the
thriving trade in erotic videos, sexy novels, books like Gina
Ogden's *Women Who Love Sex*, male strip and escort services for
women, and sex-toy tupperware parties all around Europe.

There is a sexplosion erupting in the female population, the
likes of which we have not seen since Erica Jong led us out of
the sexual wilderness and into our erotic desires too long ago.

Tired of what one woman described to me as 'the tyranny
of political correctness' that has hemmed women in erotically
over the past decade and of growing puritanical moral values,
disillusioned by a form of feminism that forced women to deny
their fantasies and erotic souls, women of all ages have risen up
in what is shaping up to be a powerful new sexual revolution.

In compiling this chapter I have spent many months travelling around the world, meeting the pioneers of the new feminist movement. The raunchy 'sex-positive activists', 'goddess
activists' or 'pleasure positivists' as they describe themselves. And
doing their workshops.

With my tongue firmly in my cheek and my finger on the
pulse I lie on the floor with a group of naked women searching for my G spot. But this, according to the goddess grrrls, is
mandatory stuff. They say female power and creativity stems
from our wombs and by unlocking our primal and sexual
energy through ritual, dance and ancient breathing techniques,
women will be empowered.

Although much of what I have seen does amuse me, I can't
hide the fact that I am also greatly impressed by a form of
feminism that does not ignore the female body. And I am

inspired by the cacophony of gutsy, sassy, outspoken new voices in the chorus.

I have, for a long time, suffered the cold shoulder of traditional feminists because my thinking doesn't toe the party line. Because I don't think it's an act of betrayal to laugh at ourselves and our own erotic contradictions. Two women equals ten opinions. We are torn, confused. We are sophisticated yet primitive at the same time. We fight for the right not to be looked at sexually whilst standing in come-fuck-me shoes and blood-red lipstick which mimics the blushing baboon bum on heat. Give me a break!

Often we don't know what we want. And far too often we want the wrong things when our hungry bodies overtake our politically correct minds. Predictably, the Sisterhood chucked a collective wettie when the story *Blokes* was first published. But as author Nancy Friday will attest, it is not uncommon for staunch feminists and strong women to fantasise about being ravaged by a Neanderthal whilst rigorously blathering about wanting the 'respect' of sensitive men.

I amuse myself with the dangerous terrain of sexual politics throughout the book. As a rampantly hormonal woman who delighted in popping her tongue where she shouldn't have on the way up the greasy pole, I know that not all women are the victims of all men all the time. Particularly when we are forced into contact with that most irresistible of creatures: the powerful male, the leader of the pack. Me Tarzan. Full of testosterone. Lord of the Jungle. Hubba hubba! Someone throw water on me!

Powerful men are women's Achilles heel. I learned this when working as a finance journalist here and in New York during the '80s and early '90s. After spending years in the company of wealthy businessmen, and inside many corporations observing the psycho-sexual dance between males and females, I can only say that before we try to legislate this treacherous and highly complicated terrain we'd do better to go back to the law of the jungle, and work forwards from there.

In the same primitive vein I believe women have far more power than we lay claim to. It is an erotic power that feminism has somehow taught us to be ashamed of.

A male friend used to say: 'Never, never underestimate the power of the muff.' Whenever he said this I would imagine the poster for a schlock sci-fi movie NO MAN IS SAFE FROM *THE KILLER VULVA* with a gigantic vagina on the rampage through the streets of New York. I loved this image. I certainly never saw myself as a victim of the male system. In fact, in the hyper-macho world of high finance, it was a definite advantage to have pussy power instead of 'a big, swinging dick'.

Yes, I know about 'the women on the factory floor' – the feminist version of my mother's guilt trip when I wouldn't eat: 'People are starving in Africa!' But to adhere to claims that all women are always victims in a patriarchal society is to vastly undermine what we have achieved. It is submitting to a clitoridectomy of the female spirit.

Not all of this chapter is about the outing of female erotic power or the insufferability of political correctness. In fact, being a hot babe, a sexually confident woman, still means a lot of pain and misery in the '90s.

For one, there's rejection to deal with. Women are now moving on men, and like men before us, we are having to deal with the harsh reality that not all *objets d'amour* are going to be available. Many of us are sitting around with bruised egos, licking our wounds, and trying to work out when 'no' really means 'no', and when it means 'yes'. And why do some dicks go down when they see a strong, instigating female?

Then there is insecurity and loneliness. The chronic over-supply of available females has meant that some women can't get men. Fearing that they have become too strong and defeminised, many are reverting to classical *femme* behaviour to attract a mate. Sadly, the growing conservative backlash is gaining international momentum.

There is still the very painful internal battle for the modern girl: to breed or not to breed. And if one finds oneself suddenly 'married with children' as I have, then how does one retain one's sexiness?

Back to politics and many women resent that we have been forced, largely by a de-sexing form of modern feminism, to walk, act and dress like men in order to survive in the workforce. We can't be pre-menstrual, menopausal, pregnant, lactating or ever fall victims to our hormones.

I want PMS NOW! to be the new feminist catch-cry. I want girls in bold lipstick and bad moods to be standing around with placards demanding the right to be moody and broody and bloody disgusting to deal with if we choose a few days a month the way men have always fallen victim to their hormones or been bloody disgusting to deal with when the mood has struck.

To body image. About 99 per cent of women I have talked to are not happy with their bodies. Those who are, are only happy for a short time, watching their gorgeous cheesecake legs assume the blue-cheese lines of varicose veins. Latest studies have shown that women are at their best from the bedroom to the boardroom when we feel good about our body image. But we are never encouraged to feel too good, for too long.

I say chuck away your glossy magazines, grrrls! They are causing enormous pain and suffering, and are undermining our potency and growing power. Chuck out the tired and useless myth that says women are bitches to work for. Chuck out the one that says all women like nice emotional, intimate sex. And let's go party.

And take this along. A road map to being female in the '90s. But be warned: I reserve the right to contradict myself. I am female. And anyone using this to navigate the confusing, conflicting, contradictory maze that is female behaviour, is guaranteed to get lost. Now, move over, boys, we're coming through!

SEXPLOSION
The sun is shining brilliantly on the water, as a group of twenty women gather in a big room overlooking Bondi Beach. We are all there to rediscover our sexuality. We are responding to an advertisement challenging us to 'unlock the sexual energy' we have all been repressing in the day-to-day grind of life.

We are not alone. All over the world women are responding to the same call. All over the world women are rising up to unleash the 'wild woman' within through courses, workshops, books and membership in exclusive clubs. A quiet revolution is brewing and those largely female entrepreneurs who are spearheading the movement are making millions of dollars out of the new wave of post-feminist sexuality.

New York-based Barbara Carrellas is one such entrepreneur. Best buddies with post-feminist porn star and multimedia sexpert, Annie Sprinkle, and the self-professed mother of masturbation, California's Betty Dodson, she has started coming regularly to Australia to spread the word.

The word is that if the '70s were about sexual liberation,

and 'zipless' escapades for women, the '80s and early '90s have been about political correctness and putting the lid on all that bubbling sexuality and eroticism. But we are coming out of the sexual dark ages again, according to the sexperts, quite literally if this 'self-loving' workshop is anything to go by.

The group of women sit trembling with fear, wondering what new level of orgasmic heights they are going to reach and if they really wish to reach them in public. I have enough trouble finding my G spot in the privacy of my bedroom let alone in the discomfort of a sexual-ecstasy production line.

But I am desperate to unleash 'the wild woman within'. The only screams coming from my bedroom late at night over the past year have been from my new baby. I've forgotten what a vagina is used for other than a baby carry bag. And don't talk to me about breasts. I'm tired of being a human milk bottle. One woman puts it very eloquently: 'To be a mother and a sexual being is very difficult. To be a mother, hold down a busy career and be a sexual creature is near impossible.'

Carrellas gently explains that she will help us reconnect with the source of our feminine power. It all sounds a little too 'New Age' for me. I nearly die laughing at the sight of the vibrators: politically correct sex-toys shaped like dolphins, whales and butterflies so you can have an environmentally-friendly climax. All toys have condoms on. In New Age thinking, even tampons should wear them.

But I'm here because I am impressed with what I have witnessed overseas. The revolution in female power is hotting up. But what has really baffled older feminists is that the pioneers and entrepreneurs behind the revolution, the once-called sex-ploiters of women, are women themselves, and staunchly feminist at that.

Madonna was only one of the new wave of women sex entrepreneurs who are making a mint out of the burgeoning new female sexual conscience they are promoting. There is a tribe of women who are sexpert buddies operating internationally as a powerful network, linked by one outstanding factor: they love sex.

Annie Sprinkle is perhaps the most outspoken. She recently caused a fracas in Australia when she presented her controversial Post-Porn Modernist stage performance at the Adelaide Festival where she turns her body into an artform and masturbates for the audience.

I spent many wonderful hours dangling out a hotel window with Annie watching the Gay and Lesbian Mardi Gras, and discussing her extraordinary creation, the workshop 'Sluts and Goddesses' being run around the world. The workshop, in Annie's words, 'helps women get back in touch with their rampant sexual desires' by encouraging women to dress up as their favourite sexual fantasy.

Annie helped Jo-Anne Baker set up The Pleasure Spot in Sydney. It is a shop which markets sex-toys to women and runs courses for women on G spot orgasms, total body orgasms and other fascinating variations on the theme. It was Baker who brought Carrellas to Australia for the workshop we are now doing.

These girls are all buddies with Veronica Vera, Wall Street stockbroker turned porn star, and now sex activist who is famous for lobbying Congress on freedom of speech. Still in America is the powerful and hugely successful film-maker Candida Royalle who is packaging porn with a more egalitarian bent.

Meanwhile in Europe the tribe includes Tuppy Owens,

outspoken London-based sex therapist and activist who pub-
lishes the *Sex Maniac's Diary* which scientifically catalogues
every sleazy and erotic club in every city of the world and
Cora, or 'Hard Cora' as she calls herself, who helped pioneer
phone-sex in Europe.

Owens says she is quite amused at how she has suddenly
become the 'darling' of feminists after years of being accused of
the heinous crime of siding with male sexploiters. She says the
younger generation of feminists are far more sexually courageous,
citing the resurgence of female interest in porn and erotica.

The Pleasure Spot's Jo-Anne Baker says: 'We are a mighty
force.' She shows me some of her sex-aids for women that she
has brought to Carrellas' workshop. There are vibrating eggs,
condoms with flowers on top in case you go off to a '70s-style
love-in, chocolate-flavoured lubricants, erotic videos, S&M
harnesses and sexy lingerie.

She says the female market is where the growth in sex-aids
is, as evidenced by the huge appetite for product in Europe,
particularly as women gain economic power.

'It's a tired old argument we've been hearing over the past
decade that all women are the victims of the sex industry and
all women are victims of male lust and that our sexuality is
purely emotional blah, blah, blah. Women are enormously sexual, sensuous beings. Blocking this energy disempowers us.'

She says, 'By learning to pleasure ourselves we can teach our
partners what we want.'

After my little chat with Jo-Anne, Barbara Carrellas
announces: 'We are going to work naked for the next two days.'
I read in the brochure that this was a workshop conducted in
the nuddy. I'd hoped there had been a printing mistake
although after thirty hours of gruelling labour I wonder how

there could be any modesty left in my body. In fact, I finally
gave birth while two burly Italian blokes with mops busily
cleaned the floor around me.

Nevertheless, I feel odd about disrobing. And I am clearly
not alone in my modesty. The women all glare at each other
apprehensively. This is out of our comfort zones. Women are
taught to be competitive with each other. To be forever assess-
ing other women's bodies and comparing them with our own
inadequacies.

Carrellas explains the philosophy behind the work: 'In
ancient times women were together in harems, in tribes, in
covens. We nurtured and supported each other while the men
were away. Now women are taught to compete with each
other, to fear each other. We are here to recapture the lost ritual of trust and support.'

It is the same rhetoric I have heard in the men's movement.
The call to ritual, to same-sex bonding. She says that the need
to play too many roles has left women confused and feeling
inadequate. The workshop will help women reconnect with
pleasure so they can feel rejuvenated by giving to themselves
for a change.

Each women in the circle is asked to talk about her view of
her body, her sexuality. I am anticipating a rather up-beat horny
sort of discussion. Instead there are stories more revealing and
naked than any physical nakedness around us.

Rose is close to seventy years old. She is the oldest member
of the group. Her skin is draped over her like a crepe curtain
full of folds and dips and yet she is the most uninhibited woman
in the room. She has not had an orgasm in over thirty years.
The reason is that her child was forcibly taken away from her
when she was a young girl. He was illegitimate in a time that

had no tolerance for such things. She has never recovered from the grief.

There are some very beautiful women in the circle, women who by any standard are shapely and sensuous. These women hate their bodies in a world where so-called women's magazines have perpetuated a negative body image. They are all sexually blocked and several can't orgasm. Others are tired and guilty from having to balance career with family obligations.

'I just don't have any energy or time for sex any more,' one woman complains as the women in the group nod. Others just feel guilty all the time about everything. It is a common theme in the room. The exhaustion felt by women. Feelings of not matching up. The sense of having to give, give and give all the time to husbands, lovers, children, bosses, businesses, girlfriends, sick or dying parents. The sense of always being judged harshly by others, and by ourselves.

The question hangs in the air as the stories intensify. What has feminism achieved over the past decade? Where is the sexual and social freedom we were promised? We are no more at peace with our bodies, our sexuality and our growing power than we were before. In fact, there seems to be enormous pain and guilt.

'We have to deal with all this anger and grief before we can move into pleasure,' says Carrellas. The morning is spent dealing with it. The nakedness is forgotten. The reason we are here is forgotten until Jo-Anne Baker opens a large bag and places on the floor twenty of the most enormous vibrators I have ever seen. Vibrators that look like they could be used on construction sites. 'God! I want to discover my vagina not excavate it,' jokes one woman as we gather around waiting for a crane to lift them into our hands.

But as I watch the women working with their bodies, as I

watch Rose exploring herself and looking transformed by the pleasure she is experiencing, I want to raise my glass to the feminist sex entrepreneurs who are challenging the old notions of political correctness and religious repression and are bravely bringing us back in touch with the sheer pleasure and joy of being a woman.

BLOKES

I have a confession to make. One that is totally ideologically unsound and politically incorrect. Though I am embarrassed to admit it, I have a secret, hidden, but powerful attraction to ... blokes.

Yes, blokes. That dying breed of male. The wonderfully archaic creature, almost as extinct as the dinosaur. He who eateth red meat. He who smoketh roll-your-owns. The kinda man who knows what goes on under the bonnet of your car. The kinda man who doesn't stand there rationally dealing with someone who insults you. The kinda man you can count on to break your heart.

I'm not saying I want one permanently. On the contrary. My husband is a most perfect specimen of SNAG (Sensitive New Age Guy). He cooks, he reads poetry and massages oils into my weary body after a hard day's work. He is magical to talk to, fair, rational, a feminist and a vegetarian. But every now and again, I have a bad craving for a bloke type individual.

I want to be knocked out by the smell of a sweaty armpit. I want my worthy opinions to be overlooked in favour of my heady perfume. I want someone to crush me with muscles used for pouring cement or mustering cattle.

Far from being threatened, my husband is amused by this trend, which afflicts other intelligent women we both know.

He says it is the post-feminist equivalent of men wanting the odd bimbo. He reckons this secret craving is what accounts for the rise in schmalzy Mills & Boon romance novels even among politically correct women, the way that many super-intelligent men buy girlie magazines or go out with the odd Tweety-bird.

He himself is given over to the occasional dribble when a leggy, busty bimbette walks into a restaurant. I've seen his eyes go glassy and his brow assume a wet, tortured look when we have visited topless beaches. I couldn't object to such lusting even if I wanted to because it is not something a wife or lover can argue with. It is a close encounter of the non-cerebral kind.

I am not implying blokes and bimbos are not intelligent but they definitely do have a different kind of wisdom. Not the bookish wisdom of the well-read, the ambitious or the fair-minded, but the wisdom of those who follow their gut instincts: into bed, into battle, into trouble.

Blokes are in touch with the raw, earthy, destructive, intense flow of testosterone in their bodies just as bimbos are in touch with the flow of oestrogen with all its horny, sensual side effects. Which make them so hopelessly appealing to people who think too much, and are chronically well-behaved, reliable, decent and God-fearing.

I would now like to devote the rest of this piece to three blokes I have loved over the past year – at a healthy distance of course.

My first attraction to a bloke lasted but an hour. It was while a girlfriend was renovating her apartment. He came with his electric power drill to open up her bathroom wall and put in a shower hose. Ah! What total bliss watching all that drilling and bashing as the tiles went flying off in different directions and sweat poured down from his ruffled hair. Blokes are so good at smashing things up. His hands were so strong I almost melted as he tugged at the concrete and threw it manfully on the ground. It brought to mind fond tribal memories of being bonked over the head with a club and schlepped into some barbarian's cave.

My girlfriend, a university lecturer, was obviously having the same reaction. We stood mesmerised as he explained the intricacies of pipes. It was the plumbing equivalent of being read T.S. Eliot. Later, as a favour (blokes will always do a lady or a 'lassy' a favour) he broke up some wooden thing outside her house with his bare hands and dragged it off.

There were plenty of things at my place I could have given him to break up and smash about but I thought better of it and went home alone.

Another favourite bloke was a car mechanic in Melbourne who saved me hundreds of dollars because he liked me. He had the heroic quality that makes women swoon. He looked under my bonnet and explained how he could recondition certain things rather than replace them. And I loved him at once as he shoved his fingers into my greasy pipes and made things right. Alas, once my mechanical thing had been reconditioned, I never saw him again.

But I have now met the ultimate bloke. The ultimate in politically repugnant, brutal maleness. I met him while out on the road doing an article on the outback.

I had to go into his farmhouse to ask for directions. He was standing in the front yard, hat pulled over his eyes, looking like the Marlboro man. He was a walking cliché, with a cigarette hanging out of his arrogant mouth. He glared at me with a look that made me glad I wasn't a homosexual Aboriginal whale.

His hands were dirty from doing something masculine with animals and you just knew you could never politely ask him to wash them if things got hot. He took me inside to see his road map. His walls were papered with guns, spears and other killing things. I felt my stomach knot with profound disapproval and my head spin from chemicals spewing up from the depth of my primordial being.

Thankfully, this close encounter of the unintelligent kind was also short-lived. He gave me directions in a gruff voice and sent me on my way.

My husband always laughs at my bloke stories, before analysing the matter with me. Though something inside makes me wish he'd grow purple with jealousy and grab me passionately in a distinctly non-New Age Sensitive, irrational, kind of way.

BOOB WORSHIP

I should have had breasts. There is no denying it. My body should have come equipped with huge boobs that bulged up through my blouse and erupted into the viewer's sight the way Dolly Parton's do.

I've often thought this over the years. The sex kitten look has always appealed to me. I have always fancied myself as a bit of a love goddess. A Sophia Loren type. A Jewish Marilyn Monroe.

I got the curves all right, but they went into the wrong spots. To put it subtly, if I walked on my hands, back to front, I'd be perfect.

I got the sort of breasts that don't keep a girl awake on hot summer nights. The kind that don't ever sag. Ever. The kind that allow you to work your way up the corporate ladder without so much as a furtive glance from male co-workers. Good, functional breasts that tuck neatly into a business suit.

I was always the envy of my bra-burning peers in the '70s while I was growing up. But I was miserable. The big, beautiful breasts that were my destiny were robbed from me by some quirk of nature that happened in the genetic swimming pool of life, and I never had a say in it.

Then one day it happened. I was having a shower and I noticed them. Bosoms. Real women's bosoms. I was pregnant.

As the months progressed these new bosoms grew fulsome and voluptuous. At night I tossed and turned as the humungous mammories rolled all over the place and got squashed under my arm. Women without breasts don't ever realise that women with breasts have to work out where to put them, particularly in bed on hot summer nights. It's a drawback, girls. A big drawback.

But though I was uncomfortable, I was blissfully delighted with my new-found fecundity. I remember the old Steve Martin joke: 'If I were a woman, I'd stay home all day and play with my tits.' That's all I did. I spent hours in the shower and in front of mirrors admiring my cleavage, tweaking my new nipples, jiggling them up and down, fondling the soft fleshy mounds that had miraculously appeared.

I spent far too long in lingerie departments buying over-sized bosom halters, and found myself worrying about the correct amount of mammary one should show through their shirt. In fact, my new tits were all I thought about. Whereas I used to just throw on a T-shirt and jeans with boyish indifference, I was now worrying about what tops I should wear. 'Hey, if ya got it, flaunt it, baby!!' I'd tell myself before deciding that it probably wasn't good to let *that* much nipple show through.

Whilst I used to just chuck on hot leather tops, tank tops, and groovy vests, I found myself wearing more shirts. And because white is a bit dull, I began wearing more floral shirts with buttons undone. My personality was slowly changing to fit my new appearance. Laura Ashley. Soft pastel. Feminine. Flouncy and light as a breast in water.

I used to be very flippant with men and competitive in a knockabout 'boys club' sort of way. Working in the macho world of finance gave me this sort of relaxed relationship. Suddenly I noticed men staring at my breasts. With all the intense male sexual attention, I found that my voluptuous personality which had developed to compensate for my snack-sized breasts, suddenly became more demure, more girlie, more coy.

I had finally become a sex kitten, breathless, excited at the sight of my own body and choc-a-bloc full of pregnancy hormones like oestrogen. But something felt very wrong. I began to miss not being able to throw myself about with tomboy glee. I knew with boobs like this I couldn't just break into a trot whilst walking along the street the way I was apt to do, or I would have knocked my front teeth out.

I began to miss myself. As my boobs grew and my hips widened into the lactating Marilyn Monroe of my dreams, I felt out of sorts. And one day I suddenly realised that I was trapped by my own titties. My boobs had me by the balls.

When I finally stopped breastfeeding and went back to work I watched those lovely breasts vanish like a special effects scene in a sci-fi movie. But the truth was I was relieved to have my old self back and I wondered why I had spent the best part of my life since puberty in a state of torment about who I wasn't.

I had been in the right body all along. Or perhaps I had grown into my body over time. At any rate we were right for each other. We had had a fabulous time together. It was a great fit. A love match. Till death us do part.

I think it is ironic that therapists' rooms are full of people trying to resolve crises with mothers, fathers and lovers. But no-one is focusing on the worst, most traumatic and unfulfilling relationship men and women seem to have: the relationship between our minds and our own imperfect bodies.

PARTY TIME

I am sitting here feeling mighty depressed because sexual harassment legislation has done irreparable damage to the office Christmas party.

Office Christmas parties can be such good value for many reasons. Firstly because you get to vomit or watch others you respect vomit – a great social leveller and a symbolic purging of the old and a hailing in of the new. You get to cry. But, most importantly, you get to look into the souls of your colleagues, the people who have surrounded you all year whose behaviour has hitherto been a mystery.

All is revealed under the hypnotic influence of the demon drink. For those sober enough to see anything that is. Facades fall away, people's true selves and feelings emerge for you in full colour.

In years gone by, before sexual harassment legislation, I gained some very interesting and invaluable insights into my colleagues.

One year in Manhattan, when I leant over to get some food, a drunk female journalist who shared the desk next to mine, prodded me in the hand with her fork, and told me she had always hated me.

A male writer called me an imperialist pig and told me he hated me. Another colleague groped me and confessed his deepest love for me.

A female colleague discovered our boss's tongue in her mouth during a heated discussion. She ran away crying. He then came and tried to share his tongue with me. As there were seven of him I didn't know what to do, so I started crying too. We were all very confused, so we all had a few more drinks.

One colleague sat down in a chair that wasn't there. I helped him up and he groped me. We drank some more and then I got a migraine and went home in a taxi and lay in bed crying until I fell asleep.

But this year, with the crackdown on politically incorrect behaviour, I will miss out on such valuable insights that hold one in good stead throughout the coming year.

Admittedly some office parties were more informative than others. One of the most useful parties occurred a few years ago and taught me that with work partners, things are often more complex than may appear.

We all were sitting around a large table. The journalist in question – a most senior and respected man – was cheerfully knocking back the grog and spinning yarns worthy of his raconteurial skills. Suddenly he was gone.

We were all surprised. No-one saw him leave. He wasn't on the floor. He wasn't in the bathroom. We searched for ten minutes, mystified. Did someone offend him?

For half an hour we discussed the strange phenomenon and then finally continued with the meal. I was in the middle of eating when I felt two hands clutch my ankles and a human form trying to climb under my skirt. I screamed and we all looked under the table. There he was, naked (except for his undies), with his shirt tied around his head and chin, smiling sheepishly up at me. He then took flight around the restaurant, amorously bellowing my name and causing a mighty fracas until tamed, dressed and placed back in his chair to a diet of black coffee. He claims no knowledge of such behaviour to this day.

Another Christmas party taught me the true intelligence of my journalistic colleagues.

On this occasion, the leading and much-respected writers of our country's news decided to conduct an experiment worthy of our noble profession: to see how many potent green drinks called dive bombers (composed of spirits and sweet liqueurs) they could consume before going unconscious.

Things got heated when a rather brutal argument erupted as to whether vomiting was or wasn't considered cheating. The matter was not resolved until the judge vomited and then we agreed it was mandatory to the achievement of the goal. I stumbled out around midnight leaving others of my esteemed, intoxicated colleagues watching in fascination. The next day it was reported in a rival newspaper that an ambulance was later summoned to collect the poisoned bodies.

One daytime office Christmas party gave me a staggering insight into a girlfriend who, after the party, invited me to Bondi Beach for a swim (to help us both chill out) and then disappeared.

She 'got lost' somewhere between our two towels which were next to each other. I was too tired and emotional to work out that she was not coming back to collect me and spent several hours in the dark, sitting in the sand crying until I realised I lived around the corner and I walked home.

Now that we have 'The Office Rules', we will all have to be good, decent and well-behaved at office Christmas parties lest some male offends some female. But it does have its benefits. Post-Christmas-party trauma is greatly reduced. I always found it hard and very unproductive to have to walk around avoiding people's eyes for the next three months and hiding behind office pillars.

THE OFFICE RULES

● Any man seen with an erection in an office setting will go directly to jail.

● Any man who thinks lustful thoughts in an office setting will receive twenty lashes lest this lead to an act of spontaneous groping of a female staff member.

● Men are to be monitored by a strobe light attached to the penis each morning as they enter the building. The device will be 'movement' sensitive.

● If a man is seen touching a female staff member for any reason whatsoever, he will be doused with petrol and set on fire in front of the entire office.

● Absolutely no drinking or tongue kissing at office Christmas parties. Men must sit separate from women and refrain from looking at women below the neck in case this leads to spontaneous breast groping.

● No more dashing into the darkroom, lunging at protruding naughty bits, or pressing genitals onto the Xerox machine to photocopy for loved ones around the office.

● Women will be forbidden from wearing come-fuck-me shoes or red lipstick in case they incite lust. Dressing in potato sacks would be greatly helpful in discouraging any unwanted 'up-risings'.

● Chocolate is to be banned from the office canteen owing to a recent report out of America that 97 per cent of people think about sex whilst eating chocolate.

OFFICE SEX

Whilst on the topic of office sex, a recent survey discovered that men in offices think about sex approximately once every half an hour. If they are under forty they think about having sex even more frequently.

This was reported in one of the women's magazines I picked up in the hairdressing salon recently.

The article told women not to be overly concerned by the fact their bosses and colleagues wanted to 'take' them in the lift shaft, up against the wall in the office library, on the filing cabinet (ouch!) or – most frequent of all – pushed against the Xerox machine. It claimed these beastly thoughts never lasted for long and rarely translated into reality.

It said the wives of these office love-machines shouldn't fret either. Unlike the female sexual fantasy, the male fantasy was superficial and transient. It had no romance to it. Men were not yearning for intimacy and warm candle-lit dinners with their co-workers. A momentary mental flash of naked thigh against a desk followed by a quick mental grope was about the extent of it.

What I want to ask the author of this article and, indeed, of the survey that inspired it is: Where? Where are all these highly potent males with bulging projectiles running around in business suits? Where are all these hot, throbbing, love-beasts with their minds full of wonderfully lusty, creative thoughts? Where are the heavy breathers with their sweaty palms who, at the very sight of a female co-worker, think immediately of 101 things to do with a Xerox? Tell me, because I'm gonna pack my briefcase and head over.

I have never in fact seen one of these creatures. Neither, I'm sure, have most of the working female population. Because, quite frankly, my experience with the male species in the workforce is that no matter how sexy and sexual a man is, the moment you put him near a desk or a computer, you've lost him.

Men get hard at the smell of ink. You can stand stark naked in front of him and do a tap dance on his desk, or do erotic eastern things with his balance sheet. But he isn't going to take the slightest bit of notice. In reality, you'd be hard pressed to find a man who had a sexual thought in the office every half-year, let alone every half-hour.

Putting a man in a business suit is like putting him in a tweed chastity belt. In all my years as a finance journalist working in various offices here and abroad and spending much time in the company of the button-and-tie brigade on Wall Street and in other business centres, I have not noticed men to be looking at anything other than their own performances.

Men in offices have but one thing on their minds: success. Sumptuous, heaving-breasted women don't even rate a mention during working hours. After hours, after the thrust and grind of nine-to-five, over a few drinks at the office Christmas party, men are more than accommodating of a woman's thrusting bosom. Indeed, they are apt to reflect most fondly on such delicacies.

But the male is an extremely competitive creature and when in a competitive environment like an office, will not allow himself the luxury – consciously or not – of being distracted from the pressing task ahead.

Which brings me to my next point. It is a female fantasy that men sit back and contemplate the wonderment of us all – anatomical or otherwise. Because, in my experience, it is females who sit around and think about being swept off to exotic places like the Xerox room or the lift. It is women who dream of moments of intense passion, not all of which include a preceding candle-lit dinner.

I know plenty of women in senior positions who have this fantasy. They yearn for the romance of a passionate embrace, for the danger of an illicit moment. One woman I know recently took the upper hand, so to speak, and threw herself against a co-worker in the office library. Apparently he was so shocked and so unable to handle the situation that he didn't come into work the next day.

Far from having a sexual thought every half-hour, he claimed later he never noticed her seductive advances. He never even noticed her, and she is one hell of a sexy, provocative lady.

When he was hovering over her looking 'longingly' at her, he was actually wondering whether or not she had prepared the research material he was using.

At a party recently, I told a female journalist that she should try working for my newspaper for a while. Her response was: 'Are there any hot, heterosexual men in your office?'

It is an absolute myth that women are the perpetual victims of male lust. Modern women are equally in touch with their sexual urges, if not even more so than men. Or at least they allow themselves more time to indulge in the wonderful world of fantasy.

Nor is it true that women's fantasies are necessarily romantic while men think only lascivious and transient thoughts. Just read Nancy Friday.

Last week I went to a female bucks night. The girls sat around all evening talking about men and sex. In stark contrast, the bride-to-be told us the next day that her fiancé and his merry band of men sat about discussing something equally exciting: the economy.

BAD MEN

My husband is appalled. I have parked myself in front of the television again to worship and ogle at TV's newest bad guy, Sheriff Lucas Buck from the series *American Gothic*.

'How can you find him attractive?' my husband laments as Buck performs a host of dastardly deeds. 'He's a pig, a monster,' he says to no avail. Seems the more piggy and monstrous Lucas Buck is each week the more I am growing attracted to him. It is beyond my control and my husband's comprehension.

'Why do women love bastards?' he asks dolefully. It is the eternal question.

He is only just getting over the confusion of *Pride and Prejudice* where each week I would drop everything, from work responsibilities to the baby, to watch the arrogant Darcy sulk, pout at the camera, sulk and then sulk some more. 'But he just sneers all the time and looks really depressed!' said husband trying to fathom the weird phenomenon of female logic.

It is pointless trying to be logical with a woman on heat. The more Darcy sneered and bared his teeth like a wild dog, the more I swooned and sweated.

Similarly I went all gooey in the movie *Dangerous Liaisons* when actor John Malkovich flashed his tongue lasciviously and malevolently at sighing virgins. As he grew wickeder, so too did I find myself sinking into the pits of lust. Sheriff Buck, like a modern-day Heathcliff, is possessed by demons and full of the horror of a tormented soul. And therein lies his profound and irresistible attraction to women.

'Why is it so,' my husband mutters, 'that women like bad men?' Quite regularly I get letters from men asking the same thing. One poor fellow recently wrote: 'I thought women wanted nice men but I keep getting dumped for some bastard.'

I agree that women get besotted with anti-heroes. Certainly my girlfriends have not failed to notice the sexual charisma of Lucas, Darcy or the smouldering eroticism of traditional clean boy Tom Cruise in *Interview With A Vampire*.

One theory touted by psychologists is that modern women are inherently masochistic. Growing up with absent fathers who were always working and never available, we were weaned on deprivation.

Hence we continue to struggle for Daddy's attention and get hooked on the sexual appeal of depriving or unattainable male figures. Even strong women fall prey to this common pattern which is compounded by the fact that nearly all of our childhood authority figures – from postmen to policemen – were male.

Sociologists reckon that this pattern was reinforced by a generation of TV shows and movies where the heroes – whether good or evil – remained emotionally distant and absent. Even the goody-two-shoes Captain James Kirk was a remote and dysfunctional workaholic who could love nothing but his ship. I recently watched an episode where he was splashed with the most potent elixir in the galaxy, the tear of some beautiful alien woman. No man had ever been able to resist its power, falling immediately in love with the woman. But Kirk was already consumed by a far greater love: *The Starship Enterprise*.

Women have learned to be forever attracted to men who cannot make emotional connections or deal with intimacy. It's the Sleeping Beauty fairytale: we are in a state of perpetual waiting for the elusive prince to kiss us and awaken us from our sleep. The impact of this on female sexuality is profound with many women I know continually needing mind games, romantic and erotic dramas associated with the unattainable male, to fuel their libidos.

Whilst acknowledging the profound effect social forces like absent fathers and remote heroes had on my generation of women (and men for that matter) I think another plausible answer can be found in the animal kingdom.

It is not bad men that women fall for so much as that bad men are often powerful men. And power is the ultimate aphrodisiac. Sheriff Lucas Buck has supernatural powers, Darcy was rich enough and elite enough to wear the sneer of arrogance. Heathcliff had risen through ill-gotten gains to rule over a large estate.

Hollywood has decided to churn out more movies and TV shows with anti-heroes in the power seat and it is casting attractive male leads like Tom Cruise and Antonio Banderas in these 'bad guy' roles to manipulate female hormonal desires.

So now we are attracted to power but have the added pleasure of battling internally with good and evil, and yielding pitifully to primordial lust.

I hasten to add that Sensitive New Age Guys should take heart. We women have wisened up over the decades. It isn't that we want to marry it or even spend an undue amount of time with powerful, bastard men or our absent fathers.

In fact, it is impossible to imagine what sort of conversation one could expect with any of these heavy, remote dudes. Hard to enjoy chatting with Heathcliff about the puppy litter he just drowned, or with Sheriff Lucas Buck about the men he just hanged. Even trying to talk to good old Captain Kirk – my childhood passion – about anything other than his ship's engine, would certainly draw a blank.

No, boys, it is merely the sexual encounter we yearn for.

The hormonal hit. We pine subconsciously to procreate with the most powerful beast in the jungle so we can make super children who will seek out new worlds and boldly go where no man has gone before. It's our biological imperative telling our personal needs to go jump.

For any bloke who doesn't get what I'm saying let me put it this way. What we feel is precisely the same instinct that makes you guys produce sperm when you set eyes on Pammy Anderson's mammaries. But would you want to marry them?

CATCH THAT MAN

The million dollar question in the '90s for women seems to be how do you get a man and keep him. I say million dollar because there's a plethora of new books and courses available to concerned women all over the world offering the so-called answer to modern-day man troubles. And those writing them are reaping in the cash.

It seems women are in the grips of a global identity crisis, unsure of how to attract men any more, unsure of how to get a man to play for keeps and to stop him from straying once you have him, in this age of ever-changing roles and new rules. Therapists and sexperts are claiming that so bad has the problem become that anyone coming up with pat answers is an instant marketing success.

The solution to the male–female dilemma may indeed be complex but that hasn't stopped thirtysomething American authors Sherrie Schneider and Ellen Fein putting out a book of mind-numbing simplicity: *The Rules*.

Based on the wisdom of someone's grandmother, it preaches a return to 1950s behaviour: play hard to get, never call him or accept a date without three days' notice, make him the centre of conversation. Despite critics' complaints that the book is the greatest backward step for feminism since the wonderbra, and a complete backlash against strong women, it is fast becoming an international best seller.

Just reading *The Rules* is enough to give anyone with even the slightest feminist leanings a heart attack.

For example: Rule 3: Don't stare at men or talk too much. Rule 5: Don't call him and rarely return his calls. Rule 6: Always end phone calls first. Rule 16: Don't tell him what to do. Rule 17: Let him take the lead. Rule 12: Stop dating him if he doesn't buy you a romantic gift...Rule 4: Don't meet him halfway or go dutch on a date. My favourite tells a woman no more than a casual kiss on the first date.

The authors write that '90s women have not been schooled in the basics of finding a husband or at least being very popular with men. This book promises to make women irresistible and desirable by teaching women how to give men the challenge of the chase.

Notions like coming on to a man, and equality, are definitely passé in this little bible of nostalgia. It is like stepping into *Pride and Prejudice* or another Jane Austen novel, and definitely indicates a harking back to the Dark Ages.

What no-one has told all the lonely women who have bought the new myth hook, line and sinker, or who are ringing up the authors at $315 an hour for a phone consultation, is that a big-mouth like me who stares at men's crotches, has always taken men to lunch and bed when it suited me, who always returns men's phone calls and who would drop everything at the drop of a hat for a good time, was never short of a date or a lover. And ended up most happily married. The challenge for men is in a woman's personality not her behaviour.

The other how-to book that most caught my eye is the hot seller *Just Between Us Girls* by Sydney Biddle-Barrows (with Judith Newman). The subtitle is: *Secrets About Men from the Madame Who Made It Her Business to Know.*

Sydney Biddle-Barrows was the 1980s version of infamous Hollywood madame, Heidi Fleiss. She once ran an up-market callgirl service in Manhattan which catered to the needs of the richest, most powerful men in the world: moguls, sheikhs, politicians.

Now she has become a mentor to middle-class women all over the country, teaching them how to prevent their husbands from straying or going to callgirls by – get ready for it – acting like callgirls.

She is harking back to that old '50s wisdom: 'A woman should be a whore in the bedroom, a chef in the kitchen…' I forget the rest but I don't think it is 'and a dynamo in the boardroom'.

According to a contact of mine in the USA, it was rumoured that Biddle-Barrows was recently invited to Los Angeles by the wives and girlfriends of several prominent film-makers and entertainment industry moguls to take a course teaching them the sexual secrets of their men. These Hollywood wives were apparently so shaken by the Heidi Fleiss saga, they desperately wanted to know how to keep their men interested.

Like *The Rules*, Biddle-Barrows' world is a very simple place. Basically it boils down to a few golden principles including letting your man be the centre of attention. She says let him be totally selfish every now and again. That's why men go to callgirls.

She reinforces that a man falls in love through his eyes. She says good grooming is a source of real power and eroticism for women. Big turn-offs include: hairspray, grey hair, too much make-up, clunky shoes, too much jewellery, outdated glasses, ratty underwear, red, 'dragon lady' fingernails, heavy perfume, nasal, high-pitched or grating voices.

Reading through all this I had a terrible sense that Ms Biddle-Barrows hadn't heard of the women's movement at all. But she redeems herself by adding that most men do like sexual self-confidence in a woman. She devotes lots of room to encouraging women to stop seeing themselves only as 'wives' and find within themselves a sense of erotic adventure, a zest for the unpredictable.

She says men love a woman who will experiment with fantasy, and her body, and new experiences. But before feminists get too overjoyed, Biddle-Barrows reminds us that men prefer blondes, in kitten-heels, who moan in bed.

I don't know how these books will line up in feminist history. I know one thing. I'm going to take Biddle-Barrows' advice and moan more in bed. 'God? Why, God, didn't you make me a blonde? Why, why... why?'

BITCHES

It is a commonly held view that women can never be trusted by other women. Your female friend will take your man the moment your back is turned. She will leer jealously at your hair, body and wardrobe as you stroll into the room. She will wish you well and secretly plot your downfall. Television shows, ads, pulp fiction and songs continue to push this view of female–female relationships.

Watch your average soap opera and the message is clear. The moment Bliss's back is turned, Caress will run off with boyfriend Brick or ex-lover Clock (yes, these are real names given to characters from daytime television). October will do some dastardly deed to undermine the happiness of sister April. Sisters are always scheming to bring misery to each other.

There are countless ways to ensure a friend's demise. A favourite in soapie land is to undo the saddle strap on the girlfriend's horse so she will fall and smash her head or lose *his* baby. Women also tend to push each other down the staircase ad nauseam. There are mud-wrestles, hair pulling, face-slapping battles and, of course, fingernail fights. Betrayal being the name of the game.

I used to find TV portrayals of women amusing but when men started to express shock at my stable of female friends, warning me that I'd be back-stabbed or de-saddled, and women started expressing fear about working for female bosses, I realised that the myth was seriously out of control. That the natural trust and empathy that I believe exists between women is being seriously undermined by false messages.

The 'bitchy girlfriend' is a myth that won't go away. And although it is a widely held truism that women will talk, chat, gossip and be matey with women around them at work or play, deep and lasting friendships between women are generally portrayed as the exception not the rule. And God forbid you should end up working for a woman.

The odd buddy movie like *Thelma and Louise* does little to debunk the myth because the lead characters are often portrayed as dysfunctional.

There was a rather offensive ad on television which showed a woman talking to her girlfriend about her latest boyfriend. When she goes into the other room, the friend takes the boyfriend's phone number, intending to call him and steal him away.

For what it's worth, I have always found intimacy and trust between women to be the norm not the exception. My girlfriends are, and have always been, my pillars of strength. My female bosses have been supportive and inspirational.

Some say I have been lucky, or just chosen well. I disagree. Linguist Deborah Tannen describes a great levelling process in woman–woman relationships called 'trouble talk' where women are apt to share the most visceral problems and details of their lives in order to create a form of bonding and intimacy.

This, she says, harks back to primitive times where women lived together in communities and nurtured and protected each other and the children, whilst the males were away killing beasts or making war.

Tannen says that most women work this way, and that even women at the top echelons of corporations or professions cannot resist the lure to meld with their sisters through the sharing of problems and perceptions. She says 'trouble talk' is a wonderful female ability to cut through rank and to level the playing field, as opposed to male talk which is usually aimed at making the talker appear one rung higher on the greasy pole.

For every woman who has tried to block another woman's rise, there are men manipulating and contriving to keep younger talent at bay. For every unpleasant, premenstrual female boss or colleague there are ten mid-life-crisis men lunging and plunging at anything they see, and throwing emotional wetties around the place.

I, for one, refuse to buy into any myth that destabilises women's natural attraction to the warmth, friendship, support and safety offered by our own sex.

TAKING IT LIKE A MAN

A few years ago, when I was a single lass, I had a very demeaning experience. The mother of all demeaning experiences in my strange, discordant life.

I met a beautiful man. A heart stopper. This was the sort of man whose female equivalent was the innocent Botticelli beauty or an ancient Greek goddess. He had both a gentle naivety and an awesome wisdom. More importantly he had long, long legs. They were always wrapped in torn jeans. He would flash those legs as provocatively as any woman, crossing and uncrossing them in front of females, slinking around the room, bending down to reveal a tight, muscle-bound tush at any excuse. And I fell desperately in lust with him.

In retrospect, the longing I felt for this man had more to do with the length of time between courses than anything else. I wanted to be in love so badly that I projected a lot of my own fantasies onto him. Reality ceased to exist. But at the time I was consumed with unrequited, uncontrollable adoration, lustful yearnings and a continual state of distraction at the mere mention of his name.

He was a close friend of my room-mate and had just broken up with his girl which meant that he often dropped in unannounced. I would rush around in make-up and stilettos from breakfast time to 2am in case he popped over.

Of course, the Universe always loves to put its finger in our little pies, so the guy would always, always, drop by when I was just coming out of the shower with wet stringy hair and red, blotchy cheeks, or as I came puffing up the driveway in daggy tracksuit bottoms after a little trot round the block to keep in shape for the impending glorious union I was expecting.

Clip-clop, clip-clop, around the kitchen for eighteen hours and then the minute I was flopping around in 'ugly' mode, presto! The doorbell would ring.

But despite the general inequity of Fate in the universal scheme of things he was obviously becoming attracted to me. He began flirting with me and popping in even when he knew my room-mate was not there. He said he loved my writing, and we spent hours pouring over my scribbles. Finally he asked me out.

Oh the dreams, the dreams and fantasies the thought of that date provoked. I stopped sleeping, tossing instead in a fitful frenzy. He would say, 'Blah, blah, blah,' then I would say, 'Blah, blah, blah, blah.' Then he would corner me against the wall and say, 'Blah, blah, blah.'

I would be blushing and demure as he held me in his strong arms and wrapped around me with his long legs.

There were other scenarios. Scores in fact. I went through every one of them from start to finish and then back again, through the long nights, so that when he made his move I'd be prepared. I did what so many girls secretly do behind the closed doors of their bedrooms. I kissed my own arm. I pashed on with my upper arm and rolled around creating the excitement that the anticipated event would bring.

It must be noted here for the record that women who haven't had sex for a while become increasingly deranged. Even grown women. Especially grown women. It is because we are desperately hungry not just for sexual release but for something far more complex. We get a sort of skin hunger. A yearning to be held and touched and made whole.

In my dreams I always imagined my *objet d'amour* begging. I was always a little reticent. Holding back provocatively as he was driven to fits of passionate despair. 'Please, please,' he would weep as I casually closed the front door.

Anyway, to cut a long, tragic story short, the date was nothing like I expected. It was a pleasant enough evening, but there were none of those long, smouldering glances that I had written into the script. And the crescendo – the last act – also did not conform to written requirements. I stood begging him to come in for coffee after he dropped me off at the front door, while he casually explained that he had to get up early for work.

Far from being discouraged, I used that as evidence of his burning passion for me. He was playing hard to get. I awarded each move of the evening with profound significance so as to keep the dream alive. By morning I felt fabulous because next time he popped in he'd say: 'Blah, blah, blah,' then attempt to 'take' me somewhere between the laundry and the front room.

He must have popped in another twenty times. He never attempted to take me at all. So one terrible, terrible day which burns like a cancer in my memory, while he was walking towards the front door, I went charging down the hall with all the fury that delusionary behaviour and unrequited love inspire and threw myself at him. I jumped with such force he was actually flung against the front door which slammed shut. I attempted date rape.

I did it because I knew he needed assistance to get over his shyness with me.

I even kept telling myself this as he began peeling my wet hands off his shoulders and saying kindly: 'Ummmm. I've patched things up with my ex. Let's be friends.'

Let's be friends. Let's be friends. The cruelest three words in the English language. 'You're very attractive but...' Oh, be still my burning cheeks! I used those words heartlessly for twenty years and the Universe had sent them back to haunt me. Karma without the Sutra.

I am telling this horrid tale for a reason. The same thing happened last week to a stunning girlfriend of mine who, in anticipation of a night of love, wore the sexiest garter belt I'd ever seen and rang me up sobbing the next day.

It happened a month ago to another lovely girlfriend who was led far further up the garden path before her partner zipped himself up and said that he didn't want to have to be forced to make a commitment so he'd rather abstain.

It's a new epidemic. Women moving on men. And having to suffer the consequences of their new-found power. Because in this exciting 'take what you want' climate for sassy women, comes the painful realisation that not everything is available.

In fact, many men are saying no to horny, sexually liberated women – because of fear of commitment, because of huge availability of stock, or simply because some conventional dicks don't respond well to strong, raunchy women taking control.

And it's a hard pill for women to swallow. More responsibility, more assertiveness and instigating, means more rejection, as it has always meant for men.

Some women claim it has made them stronger. Like men, there are those with a competitive spirit who welcome brick walls. It makes them climb higher and harder.

But others who are a little frailer in the ego department, talk of shattered morale, of feeling blinded by pain. Because women of my generation were not socialised to be rejected, we are still floundering with the taking-it-on-the-chin mentality.

In fact in the treacherous new terrain we are conquering, I think it is going to be a long time before women fully understand the meaning and impact of those ever-brutal words: *take it like a man*.

MACHO BABES

Something intriguing is happening to our cushier suburbs. These havens of opulence, these haunts of the rich and famous with their fabulous harbour views, boutiques and women in

haute couture, are rapidly turning into wild, uncharted bush-
land. Smooth bitumen is turning into rugged dirt track. Harm-
less suburban trees are transmogrifying into dangerous,
man-eating plants.

Well, it's a theory. How else does a normal, logical-thinking
person explain the sudden epidemic of four-wheel drives and
jeeps with names like 'Cherokee' and 'Warrior' that have taken
over the roads in the exclusive Eastern Suburbs of Sydney and
Melbourne and the wealthier parts of other national cities?

Move over the Leyland Brothers. It seems it is no longer
safe to sit outside a school at home-time unless you are barri-
caded in a vehicle more intimidating than the Pope-mobile. At
3pm, the streets outside Sydney's private schools are clogged
with Range Rovers and monster jeeps with huge tyres. I know
that children can become extremely hungry by the end of
school but have they turned savage? Is this *Lord of the Flies* revisited? Do we need protection from untamed kids brandishing
notepads and biros like Zulu warriors descending on a village?

Parents will often claim that it is for the children's safety that
they buy these huge, throbbing machines. But independent
assessments have found jeeps no safer on the roads than ordinary cars, in fact they can more easily roll.

Perhaps parents are worried about what dangers lie in the
five-kilometre stretch along the harbour-side from school to
home: tigers, wild game, a herd of wildebeests on the charge?
Maybe a few terrorist gangs ready to turn Australia's inner suburbs into a new Bosnia. Perhaps mothers may have to drive
through deadly swamps? Or navigate deftly over sand dunes?

Clearly these creatures are the new yuppie equivalent to the
long fronted car. Now you are big, big vertically in these whopping, pulsating pieces of machinery. The big irony of the big car

is that it is mostly women behind the wheel of what can only be described as the most overt form of penis envy I've ever seen.

Women go tearing around in these bully mobiles, terrorising smaller cars, clogging the roads and feeling powerful and potent in their 'my dick's bigger than yours' machine. This is the rich-bitch equivalent of the career grrrl. The domestic doll's answer to the briefcase or corporate shoulder-pad. The stay-at-home wife's version of pussy power.

Well-kept babes are buying well-paid women's fantasies – which are based on well-paid male fantasies – about escaping the pampered life and roughing it. But a quick peek into these bully jeeps reveals that most female drivers have never seen a dirt track in their lives. The long, red nails that clutch the over-sized steering wheel, coiffured blonde or brunette hair, thick red come-love-me lips, gold chains, haven't been windblown since the last blow-wave.

Suburban mums look so ridiculous trying to hoist themselves into their Range Rovers with their shopping bags whilst not breaking off a stiletto heel. One friend ventured that bored housewives liked bully jeeps because the height enabled them to perve on men's crotches as they drove past.

To be fair, it is clear the massive roo bars are an advantage if you are about to encounter a rush of drought-starved kangaroo or emu running onto the road from Bondi Beach. It certainly was an advantage to a super-bitch the other day who tried to intimidate me into moving from my parking spot before I was ready, by almost ramming me.

The fact is that many of the urban cowgirls who own these four-wheel drives can't handle their multi-functional gear sticks any more than our narrow suburban roads can handle them. But they feel fantastic dressing up in drag. They feel powerful and wild and free.

Perhaps a clever entrepreneur should open an equivalent to the car wash in the cushy suburbs – the 'poser' wash. This will be a place you can drive your rich-bitch jeep in to get mud thrown against the roo bar, and dead insects plastered in prominent places on the windscreen to make it look like you've really been out the bush. Ah . . . boys and their toys.

THE SMELL OF SUCCESS

Of all the romantic things that can happen to a woman, having something of worth named after her by a creative man, or becoming the subject of a work of art or poem, ranks most highly.

Most women can only clench their teeth in envy at the lucky ladies whose names head up the love songs we hear on the radio, or who – like the great Mona Lisa – have faces that adorn great paintings to peer, for eternity, out at the world.

Having a perfume named after you is possibly the most romantic of romantic things that can befall a maiden.

Well, I too have had something special named after me. It isn't quite a painting, but a work of art, nonetheless. It isn't quite a perfume but it is linked to the olfactory system. One of my former beaus, in a moment of great passion, once named a shoe after me. The Ruth Shoe.

The Ruth Shoe arose because the fellow, who designed and made shoes, commented that my feet were apt to smell in summer. To avoid the unpleasantness that followed the removal of my shoes on hot summer nights, he designed a shoe which had discreet holes all along the sides to act as ventilation. Basically, to help the pong escape before I arrived at his door.

The Ruth Shoe, advertised on the box as 'A shoe for the elegant woman who wants to dance all night and remain elegant', did very well that season. In fact it sold out. At the time, I was delighted to have my name jealously bandied about shoe shops around the country although in retrospect, a song or a passionate perfume called 'Ruthless' would have done me better.

I was surprised the clever Ruth Shoe did not emerge the following season. I guess it had something to do with the fact that my beau had already moved on to more delicate hooves.

Which brings me to my main point. I was forced to think about my feet last weekend after I read an article about self-loathing. An article in a women's magazine discussed how we are all prone to dislike ourselves at times and engage in rather brutal self-hatred. This usually manifests itself in obsessive dwelling on a particular part of the body which one chooses to blame for one's miseries or to use as the body's whipping boy.

The story told how the world's most beautiful women deeply resented parts of themselves. Jerry Hall allegedly hates her 'crossed front teeth'. Michelle Pfeiffer is reputed to have said that she can't understand what men see in her. 'I have a face like a duck. At school I was teased so ruthlessly, I'd run home weeping.'

In the article it claims that Kim Basinger hates her mouth because it is 'too big' and 'ugly', while Jessica Lange apparently hates her nose which was injured when she fell against a parking meter as a child. Daryl Hannah sees herself as a gangly bean pole and hates her crooked nose, stringy hair and blotches. Even Katharine Hepburn in an old TV interview said she could not see herself as particularly attractive.

These women all blame their physical imperfections for the various sadnesses and failures that have dogged their lives.

As I was reading, my feet started tapping nervously under the table. They knew what was coming. 'Shut up,' I yelled down at them because my ill-shaped feet have always worn most of my inner hostility. In truth, I blame my strange feet for much of what has gone wrong with my life. They have slowed me down at each turn.

I have hated my feet since I was a child. At first everyone used to make a big fuss of me because of my 'cute, fat, little feet'. Later, my legs grew longer but my feet stayed the same. Which was still okay because Mum didn't have to buy me new shoes every year like other mothers did, so everyone remained really happy with my cute feet.

But by sixteen, my feet hadn't really grown much at all. They were, and have since remained, the smallest, fattest feet of anyone I know. Because they are so small and have had to carry a substantial weight, they have completely flattened at the base. So they are short, fat, flat feet. They are as wide as they are long. 'Duck feet, duck feet,' they used to sneer at school.

While other teenage girls yearned for big blonde Farrah Fawcett hair, and boys yearned for huge dongs, I used to watch other people's big feet with envy. At parties, I'd secretly wear my mother's shoes, stuffing socks into the toe area to keep the shoes on. I looked good but could never walk or dance.

And why my feet began to pong in summer was because I could never find a shoe that fitted properly. Any shoe small enough to fit length-wise, was always too narrow and squashed my foot to death in the sweltering mini-coffins I wore.

I spent my youth shuffling about in cramped shoes until one happy day when, just as Destiny brought the big-toothed Jerry Hall the impossibly bigger-toothed Mick Jagger to make her feel better, Fate brought me a beau who knew about shoes.

He told me I could have lasts made to fit my own foot size – which changed, if nothing else, the speed at which I moved through life.

As I now read the article on hated body parts something dawns on me. Perhaps my feet, rather than slowing me down in life, have actually carried me on to success in the same way the plethora of insecurities seem to have driven these starlets forward.

After all, I was always so worried people would look and laugh at my feet, I worked very hard to keep their attention focused on everything above the knee, spending much time on the art of conversation and humour. I developed my personality, and social skills figuring that if anyone had time to get down to my feet, I wasn't doing my job.

Do I owe it all to you, my fat, little, squashed dumplings? My Achilles heels? And could it be our impediments are, indeed, always our advantages, because they drive us on to better things?

PMS NOW!

'Women are strange, mysterious creatures,' my husband mutters as he wanders around from room to room. 'So, so irrational. So unpredictable. All that stuff going on inside them,' he moans under his breath.

It is not the first time I have heard him bleating. It's that time of month again and he knows that his beautiful, gentle wife so warm and fluffy, his 'little butter-ball' as he likes to call me suddenly becomes the three-eyed monster from the black lagoon, the horned beast, a grizzly, foul-tempered little troll – horrible one minute, deranged the next.

He ruminates loudly about the time I rammed my car into another car just because the driver was attempting to back into a parking spot I had seen first. He mumbles about the time he had to pick lumps of food off one of our treasured paintings after the roast chicken flew across the room during one of my PMS (premenstrual syndrome) turns.

He knows too well the telltale signs – those puffy eyes, swollen and aching limbs, everything being done in slow motion with lots of moaning and complaining. He knows well the frustration of glaring into the vacant eyes of a pea head who can no longer tell left from right, the depressions, hyper-sensitivity followed ultimately by the emotional avalanche from hell.

'My goodness, could it be that time of month already, butter-ball?' he says sweetly, whilst running to find cover.

My fellow sisters hate me talking this way. True feminists are not allowed to admit we get PMS in case men find out that we are female and hence hormonally different from them. They will then use it against us in the workforce to put up glass ceilings, wooden doors, concrete road blocks, ten-tonne mountains, mile-high fortresses and a banana skin. But girls, girls, girls – let's get real!

It doesn't affect your career progress to have the occasional 'off' day or two every month any more than it affects a bloke to have his mid-life crisis very publicly or fall victim to his testosterone urges of aggression or passion – to come back from lunch every other week sloshed to the eyeballs. But it certainly does affect your relationships at home.

And it's high time we started telling the truth. Pre-menstrual women are yucky, yucky creatures who bark like wild beasts one minute and weep uncontrollably the next. The only mitigating factor is that the cocktail of hormones gone wild does something fantastic to the female libido. Hot sex is on the cards – for the man brave enough to risk mating with a tarantula, that is.

As a gift to my long-suffering husband, and all the confused husbands and boyfriends of the world, I am going to try and explain why so many of us become hateful little trolls before our periods.

From speaking to my gynaecologist I have discovered that the answer lies in understanding women's hormonal cycles. Recent studies into menopause have been particularly useful in unlocking the mysteries of female behaviour.

It is now widely believed that menopausal women become deficient in oestrogen. As a result, feelings of well-being and energy can disappear and many women can become mighty grumpy, particularly those having regular hot flushes. Others say they feel permanently confused, especially in relation to maths or direction.

Let me give an example. Last year I was picked up from the airport in Melbourne by an older female friend of mine. We travelled swiftly down the Tullamarine Freeway without a hitch. But when we hit town, a strange thing happened.

My friend, who has driven back and forth from the airport for many years and who has lived in Melbourne for most of her fifty years of life, suddenly turned and went the wrong way.

'Where are we going?' I asked, astonished. 'I thought you were taking me to the Eastern Suburbs.'

'We are going to the Eastern Suburbs,' she assured me, continuing to drive to the outskirts of the city which lead, ultimately, to the Hume Highway and back to Sydney.

I sat pondering our fate. I started to argue, but was told to stop being bossy. So I remained silent as the streets grew foreign and the surrounding landscape more unfamiliar and confusing. Finally a sign flashed into view which indicated that we were, in fact, heading back towards Sydney.

'What's happening here?' my friend asked in shock. 'They've changed the city.'

'No,' I said gently. 'You've just lost your way.' Then she pulled over, put her head in her hands and began to weep. 'I'm so confused,' she sobbed. 'I'm going through menopause and I've suddenly lost all sense of direction. Some days I can't make out where I am.'

Apparently it is quite common for menopausal women to experience blinding confusion due to disturbed chemical cocktails. But what has all this got to do with PMS? As with menopause, pregnancy or breastfeeding, there are huge hormonal fluctuations that occur during the menstrual cycle, with no less than seven hormones involved.

Some of the hormones that are necessary for feeling okay are in very low supply by the end of the cycle. As with menopause, oestrogen is apparently at its lowest ebb just before menstruation. Meanwhile it was recently argued in England that a woman who committed murder, was not producing a hormone or chemical vital for inhibiting violent impulses in humans, at this time of month.

Like my poor menopausal friend, I too have noticed that I suffer from a similar geographical dyslexia on the roads at 'that' time of the month.

Experts in the United States and Canada have recently completed a series of tests which they claim show the direct correlation between hormones, menstrual cycles, and the ability for the human brain to negotiate spatial relationships, directions and solve numerical problems.

Meanwhile it has been shown that when menopausal

women are given oestrogen and other hormones in the form of hormone replacement therapy (HRT), many cheer up. The woman I just described claims that after being on HRT for a few months, the feeling of foggy-headedness was replaced with clarity of vision and a sense of exuberance.

There are many in the medical and psychiatric fields who are openly sceptical that PMS exists, saying that it's all in the head. This is largely fuelled by the fact that not all women metabolise hormones at the same rate, and hence not all women suffer PMS to the same degree. Similarly, not all menopausal women have the same symptoms.

Some lucky women don't suffer PMS at all, but most women I know have some disruption and are simply too frightened to own up to it.

Those more enlightened researchers and thinkers such as my gynaecologist look at the treatment of menopausal women and make the connection. It is increasingly evident that many women are the victims of their hormones as many men are now believed to be.

Does this information help anyone? It can and will when women are prepared to stop hiding from the feminist thought police and start demanding more medical and scientific investigation into what it means to be a woman – in the fullest hormonal sense of the word.

WHEN MOTHER COMES TO STAY

P.S. This story was written just before I met my husband.

A week before my mother comes to stay I have a recurring nightmare. She walks into the apartment I have just bought and stands in the middle of the room with a disapproving look on her face. The apartment isn't much to look at inside – your standard small flat, basic furniture. But the view is something quite stunning. Overwhelming, in fact.

I drag her over to the windows to show off the panorama but heavy curtains have suddenly appeared. And they won't open. I am desperately trying to explain the view of the ocean and cliffs outside the window as I yank at the rigid material, but she continues to look around the average flat, disappointed.

Eventually she walks away.

I know the dream is about trying to justify to her what I have become, and the decisions I've made in my life. I know it's about wanting her approval. I know also that with our parents, those curtains never really open, no matter how hard we try to reveal the beauty and success behind them.

Before Mum arrives I do everything she has taught me to do. I do a thorough shop, I vacuum and dust till every last speck is removed. I clean behind the stove and the toilet. No hairs on the floor. No dirt behind the sink (or my ears). My flat is 'so clean you could eat off the floor' – the boast of my family. Normally you could eat off my floor all right, so much food about.

It has taken me all of my thirtysomething years to break away from Mother. To learn that I am not her. That I don't have to have the same feelings, values, ideas. It has taken me all that time to stop feeling guilty that I'm not her.

And so she lands, and the tour of my life begins. No heavy curtains mysteriously appear on the windows of my flat. The sun has turned on a glorious treat and the views are sparkling as she makes the appropriate 'wow' type noises.

For an hour she is forced to watch all my TV appearances on tape and make the appropriate 'wow' noises, and look at every acquisition of mine and make the appropriate 'wow' noises. And only when I am content that she is truly, undoubtedly, impressed with what I have done with my life, and that my career has exceeded all of her wildest expectations, and that everyone back home is suitably impressed, do I settle back onto the couch relaxed.

But while the waves crash loudly outside my open window the mysterious curtain starts creeping down, down...

'Did you know your old friend Shelly got married last week?' Mum asks innocuously.

I feel my gut tense up. 'I haven't spoken to Shelly for twelve years, Mum. She's not a friend.'

'Well, anyway she got married.'

'That's nice, Mum.'

'And your cousin Sam just got engaged. Did you know?'

'No, Mum. But that's very nice.'

That curtain is beginning to stick to the window.

'And your friend from school, Kathy. Well she just had a baby.' I begin pulling at the curtains. In my head I'm crying: 'Look at my view. Look at my achievement. Mum, can't you see it?'

Instead I say: 'Mum. I don't remember Kathy. I'm not really interested in these people.'

'Well, I thought you may like to know. Oh, by the way, my friend Betty's daughter just had a baby girl. I went to their wedding. It was lovely.'

You can clean your cupboards. You can clean your floors. But you can never sweep away the truth. It sits like a large stain in the centre of the room. In the centre of my life. In the centre of my relationship with my mother.

At my age she already had more children than I've had hot

breakfasts. There is a home movie of Mum, aged twentysome-thing, with several fat babies hanging from her arms. She would have had more if she had the strength.

'You work so hard,' she says, turning over the pages of a magazine I recently appeared in. 'You seem...well, I don't mean to be critical, but...obsessed with your career.'

'Yes, Mum,' I sigh. 'I am obsessed with my career.'

'Will it make you happy in the end?'

'It makes me happy now.'

'But what about love?'

'I am in love. I love my life, my work, my writing, the creativity, the independence that comes from it, my friends.'

'But it's not healthy. It's dangerous to be so obsessed with your career. It's not balanced. If you lose your job you'll be devastated.'

'If women lose their husbands or get divorced they are dev-astated too. But you wouldn't tell me it's dangerous if I loved my husband or child to the point of obsession.'

Silence.

'But you don't have a child and a husband, so it's a moot point isn't it?' she snaps, turning away from me.

The ocean continues to lap against the cliff outside my win-dow. The window in the apartment I bought and renovated by myself from the fruits of my work. Every column is like a child for me, created and nursed and worried about. Every TV seg-ment, every speech is born from my labour. I don't feel empty for not having had a baby. And yet I feel guilty for not feeling empty.

I look at Mum's face – the confusion, the sadness, her love for me, her worry – and I feel an overwhelming need to pla-cate her. 'I will get married and have children. I do want those things. But not just yet. I'm so young. There's plenty of time.

There are so many things I want to do first, to learn, to experience. Today, women can have everything.'

For a moment I think she sees the vista from the window – the great expanse of my life stretched out before me. But the words 'Down Syndrome' suddenly emerge from her lips, along with 'higher risk...old eggs...tired body...biological clock...' She says sadly, 'You'll be a very unfulfilled woman...'

Like my dream, she walks off towards my tiny kitchen as I stand tugging desperately at the heavy curtain that has suddenly descended on my life.

THIRTY NOT OUT

My husband has carted me off to the doctor. He is really worried. Something serious had started to happen to my hormones over the past twelve months. Something really serious indeed.

Despite the sleep deprivation that comes with having a small child, despite the endless hours of work, despite discussions about bills and cars breaking down and leaking pipes, my libido is shining through. In fact, it is shining through like a floodlight.

To put it delicately, I have loving on the brain. Probably twenty-four hours a day. 'You are turning into a sex addict,' my husband quivers as he reads an article on the topic in a women's magazine. Sex addict is the new hip term for the terminally excited.

In the old days when you got too horny they called you a stud, a nympho, promiscuous or just plain old lucky. Now people who think about sex too much or who want it too much are locked away in an institution and forced to confess: 'I loved five women today,' or 'I loved only one man, but I loved him every fifteen minutes for two years solid.' Sort of like an Alcoholics Anonymous for the sexually deranged.

The doctor is very amused by my anxious husband. He grins at me as he answers. 'No, your wife is not a sex addict or abnormal in any way. I am happy to announce that you are the proud owner of a regular thirtysomething female.'

'Females in their thirties,' he says laughing, 'are at their sexual peak. They are like eighteen-year-old boys. Bombarded with libidinous urges, overcome with hormones. Flushed with excitement all day, every day. They're terrific,' he says beaming from ear to ear. 'I wish I had one...'

He is right. Thirtysomething females are everywhere, running riot around the streets. Bizarre hormone cocktails swirling in their bodies like adolescent schoolboys. Like smouldering volcanoes always threatening to explode in a gush of molten lava.

They are the girls with breasts sprouting out of tight vests. They are the lunatic people who go to Chippendales and bark sexual obscenities at the toy-boys on stage. They are the women who crotch-watch men from cafe windows, who run off from marriages into the waiting arms of illicit lovers or to buy huge, plug-in vibrators. They are my friends.

Indeed if you hear the hum of an electronic device for more than an hour at a time from next door, and your TV goes crazy from the static, you can be certain a female in her thirties lives there.

Thirtysomething females are the burgeoning new class of females going to male escort agencies. They are not Revolutionaries; they can't think straight enough to be making a political statement about sexual freedom.

Most men don't know what to do being married to a thirtysomething female. My husband tries tactfully to ignore me when I spontaneously wolf-whistle out of the car window. He describes it as 'hell on earth'. But the sex doctor consoles him by telling him that he only has to put up with this for a few more years then I will plunge headlong into that dank, dark state called menopause.

Why is there such a surge in thirtysomething females? Or if there has always existed this rampant species, then why have they suddenly become so visual? Where are they all coming from, my husband wants to know.

Indeed, there have been thirtysomething females since the dawn of time. But in the '90s they are not stuck at home with thirteen children, too tired to even realise they have a libido. They are in the workforce with kids in daycare when it hits. When the truck of love runs over their heads. They have all their options open so to speak, looking great well into their forties, many with economic freedom.

By why now? my husband laments. Why from ages thirty to forty and not at a time better suited to men? The doctor explains that this is the female body's last hurrah before menopause. Nature's last attempt to get women out and pro-creating en masse before the final capacity dries up.

According to some therapists, this fuzzy-headed hormonal time may well account for the huge swing in infidelity amongst married women. The thirties are a very vulnerable time for married women and can be likened to the male's mid-life crisis.

Recent statistics confirmed the degree of the problem. Only last month a major survey presented to the Association of European Psychiatrists in London confirmed that women's libidos were on the rise as men's were declining. From ages twenty-eight to thirty-five men's libidos dropped eleven per cent whilst women interviewed showed far more sexual desire at ages thirty to forty than at age twenty.

The session is over. But my husband won't leave. 'Please

don't make me go home, doctor…I can't take any more,' he says, clinging to the chair, just another desperate male voice crying out for mercy and understanding in a world suddenly brimming with thirtysomething females.

LETTERS

Dear Ruth,

Forget about plunging into 'dank, dark menopause'. What about Hormone Replacement Therapy? No more fear of pregnancies or children popping unexpected into bedrooms. Sex is great, better than it has ever been. I thought I was frigid until I reached this age.

AVID READER, NSW

Dear Ruth,

If, as a woman in her thirties, you are finding the constant urge to have sex a bit overwhelming, just wait till you hit forty!

MRS S., BRISBANE, QLD

Dear Ruth,

I am now in my late forties and the great majority of my friends the same age, all agree that this is the most sexual time of our lives. My husband, middle fifties, pretended to be impotent, but was having an affair with a woman who was also in her fifties (and gone through menopause). So I guess there is no end to this sexual drive for women. I am sure you will receive a lot of mail from older women who will assure you that you don't have a monopoly on sex in the thirties.

J., SHAILER PARK, QLD

Dear Ruth,

I believe there is one real reason why men stray. Because females seduce them. In my sixty-odd years of my sexual activity, I had sex with sixty-nine separate women. In all these, not once was I the hunter. In each case, the females seduced me to have sex with them. And I co-operated, for after all, I am human.

ANON., RENMARK, SA

Dear Ruth,

I'm sick of women saying to me 'all men want is sex'. I'm in my forties, and after three relationships I'm still looking for that man who only wants sex. None so far can keep up with me. All I want is a man who can respect me and have fun – and whatever the time of the day, enjoy sex.

MS K., QLD

Ruth Ostrow,

When are you girls going to wake up and realise that most men do not like assertive and/or feminist women? No real man is going to put up with being told what to do and be continually criticised by any woman. While I agree women are entitled to equal pay and equal rights, we are not going to tolerate outspoken loudmouth women. Try being more like your mothers, waving goodbye to your men when they go to work and greeting them at the door when they come home.

JOHN, MOSMAN, NSW

Dear Ruth,

Of course there is a very sensible reason for all adolescent females to learn to 'pleasure' oneself. The fastest, most effective way to relieve ovulation and period pain as well as PMS is orgasm. Also great for insomnia! It is faster-acting than Panadol, no chance of allergic reaction, without the need of a man to operate the mechanics and is the epitome of self-empowerment.

ANON., MUNDINGBURRA, QLD

Dear Ruth,

I had been a faithful wife for twenty-seven years. During this time not once did I have an orgasm. Then I met a wonderful man who treats me like a delicate flower. Every time we have made love I have orgasmed, and oh, how I have orgasmed. Pure bliss! Ladies, don't ever think that sex is a waste of time and that the man should get all the enjoyment!

CONTENTED, MACKAY, QLD

Dear Ruth,

You asked us to share our fantasies. As a feminist and career woman, I have always felt uncomfortable about my fantasies to be dominated, tied up and forced to submit. In reality, I am disgusted by such acts, yet privately they excite me. I am interested to hear if other women have the same conflict.

ANON.

Dear Ruth,

I was one who did all the special things for my man, but I now feel uncomfortable about being naked in front of him. Since breast-feeding, my bust size has gone right down, and when your partner says things like, 'your tits aren't big enough', it can really hurt and make you feel quite inadequate. If it weren't for men being so paranoid over women's bodies, then we'd all feel a little more comfortable with the way we look.

KERRY, BANKSIA PARK, SA

Dear Ruth,

A year or so after my husband passed away, a concerned girlfriend of mine – knowing I was frustrated with normal sexual urges, but not wanting me to be with another man – introduced me to a Japanese vibrator. The pleasures and enormous satisfaction are unbelievable, enabling me to at last get on with my life. There must be thousands of women out there in similar situations as myself.

ANON., BURLEIGH HEADS, QLD

CHAPTER TWO

SWEATY BLOKES:
A user's guide

FROM a social and sexual point of view, the 1990s have not been kind to men. Many, it seems, are in the grips of a global identity crisis as manifested by the new social phenomenon called 'The Male Headache'. As a new twist on an old theme it is men, not women, who are turning to their wives and partners in bedrooms across the world and uttering the immortal line: 'Not tonight, dear, I've got a headache.'

According to sex therapists and researchers, the Male Headache or 'Not Tonight, Josephine' syndrome, has grown so acute over the past few years it is having a crushing impact on the way men and women relate.

Several of the sex therapists I spoke to in Australia confirmed findings from abroad – that men en masse are saying 'no' to sex, and frustrated women are bombarding them with complaints about tired or reluctant husbands and partners.

Contrary to popular myths about women not wanting as much sex as their husbands, it is married females who are now presenting as the highest growth-rate statistic in infidelity, according to Ian Macdonald, Executive Director of Relationships Australia in Queensland, and marriages everywhere are beginning to feel the strain.

Theorists are at a loss to explain the phenomenon. Some maintain that changing gender roles are having a far greater impact on men than is commonly presumed. Some say men are feeling intimidated by women's burgeoning economic power. Others claim that women want too much of men. That the pendulum has swung too far off course and this is creating performance anxiety in males.

Women want men to behave like vibrators and keep going, when really it is men's biological imperative to ejaculate, says one of my sources, sex therapist and original thinker Dr Sandra Pertot. 'Women's expectations of men have become unrealistic and this is contributing to the problem,' she tells me.

'Bob', a patient of a sex therapist I interviewed, agrees he is suffering performance anxiety at home. 'I do feel horny but not as often as my wife. But she makes me feel so bad about it, I end up avoiding sex altogether.'

Other men just feel resentful in general. A letter I received recently from one of my readers gave a brief insight into male rage. 'Given that the vast majority of men can only have one orgasm per act of intercourse, and many women experience multiple orgasms, it is obvious that men get a raw deal, particularly with the amount of effort it takes to get women into bed,' he says.

Meanwhile there are other great anxieties for males in the '90s which I examine in this chapter. The number of men rushing off to impotency clinics is on the rise, if nothing else is. More alarming is the number of men rushing off to the new breed of 'dick doctors', as they are jokingly called, having penis extension operations.

But just as women have been sorely wounded by the need to remain ever slim and youthful, I feel men have been severely damaged and disempowered by the emphasis in society on penis size and how long a male should keep it up. I think it's shameful that women are so vocal about being trapped in a beauty myth but rarely do we speak out to allay men's equally painful misconceptions about their penises.

Throughout my writings, I have attempted to put men out of their misery by announcing that for at least one horny female 'It ain't what you got but the way that you use it'. Interesting to note that following publication of several articles I have written on this topic, I received a tremendous amount of mail from men, pouring out their gratitude and passing valuable information on to other men.

Well-endowed Mr R.R. from Perth wrote: 'I have heard the female cry "bigger is better" many times before but have yet to meet a female who really enjoys having intercourse with an "enviable size penis". Most times, if not always, their eyes are far bigger than their vaginas.'

Another West Australian reader, Anon. from Sorrento, says: 'I am a man with a ten-inch member. My wife was the only woman I ever met who could actually accommodate the length. She maintains that the banging on the bottom of her cervix is a pain she enjoys because it triggers a different type of orgasm. But had I not met my wife, I think my blessing would have been more of a frustration.'

The '90s has also been a time of profound confusion for men in terms of interpersonal relationships. Men genuinely don't understand what women want of them. Perhaps that's because we are so confused about what we want. Socialised with one set of values, coming of age with another, we want bastards who do the ironing and talk to whales.

Glenn Wallace from Sanderson in the Northern Territory, one of my favourite and most prolific letter writers, puts it thus:

'Now, according to your column we are supposed to be a refined combination of both a Neanderthal who clubs his woman on the head and drags her into his cave by the hair – but also a Sensitive New Age Guy who assumes the responsibility for her having an orgasm and turns emotional if she didn't enjoy it as much as he did. Of course men haven't changed since the days of the cave dweller. We are still totally mystified and perplexed as to just what women want from us in a relationship.'

It all sounds very woeful for men, but before women start taking out their hankies and weeping, they'd better read the rest of the chapter. Visiting men in their natural habitats I have discovered that boys will always be boys – hot, crude, naughty and bursting with testosterone. And I, for one, love them for it!

DOES SIZE COUNT?

Does size matter? I was just reading an article in a New York magazine about a fellow who spent his entire inheritance so he could join an elite group of men in America who have humungous penises. Apparently before the operation his member was working very well, his girlfriend content. But because she only orgasmed every other time, the misguided fellow thought he was to blame and instead of talking to her, went to see a doctor to have his schlong enlarged.

Unfortunately the operation left the man considerably worse off, according to the report, sparking possible litigation.

If the story was not enough to make any feeling human being squirm in their chair, a picture accompanying the article was worse. It showed a bloke with a ten pound weight hanging off his member.

Believe it or not, this technique – which sounds like a modern-day version of torture on the rack – is gaining increasing attention across the US as a way of creating a longer schlong or at least preventing shrinkage. Apparently you are supposed to wear the weights or dumbbells for several hours a day: Ooooh!

After speculating about how any man would be able to find underpants big enough to cover the weights (Is that a ten pound dumbbell in your pocket or are you just glad to see me?) I decided that enough is enough. It's time to tackle the delicate issue of size and performance head-on, so to speak.

From the letters I have been getting, it seems that most men are not certain the degree to which size, and length of time they can sustain an erection, really matters to women. The saddest part of the letters is the shame and torment buried between the lines. 'I'm too embarrassed to ask,' wrote one twenty-three-year-old man after asking *me* to tell him if his girlfriend was satisfied with his penis.

Meanwhile the plethora of impotency clinics now advertising every week has many men, even the most sturdy egoists, questioning their potency. Dr Michael Lowy of the Australian Centre for Sexual Health at St Luke's Hospital says: 'While it is wonderful these clinics are available to help men with erection problems, the down-side is that it makes many men doubt themselves.

'The promotional advertising for these clinics reinforces the idea that successful sex is solely dependent on the performance of the man's penis, which is false and just plays up to men's deepest fears and feelings of inadequacy.'

So before men rush off to buy dumbbells, or to clinics to inject their penises so they can stay erect all night, here are women's views on male performance as written about in girls' glossy magazines (which men rarely get to read) and as told to me by countless women over the years.

Myth: size matters to most women. Wrong. Long schlongs are very aesthetically pleasing to women, I won't lie about this. I'm going on the record along with self-confessed lesbian activist Camille Paglia who recently wrote a surprising article in praise of the fulsome male member. But it all amounts to nothing much.

The size of a man's penis is, I would say, as relevant as a woman having large and sensual breasts. Big boobs are great. Lovely to look at. But the majority of us females work just fine without them. Which leads me into the second greatest myth of the twentieth century: *that larger penises give women more pleasure.*

No, no, no, no and no. Anatomically inaccurate.

Every vagina is different. And as such responds to different stimulus. One of the smallest men I knew was fantastic in bed because he managed to hit my G spot. As we girls say, 'It ain't the size of the prize, it's the angle of the dangle,' honey!

Some men with very big members lose erections early because of the amount of blood it takes to carry the hefty load. However, this is not always the case. Some long ones hit the cervix of women who have low-lying wombs. Some women absolutely love this sensation. Others hate it with equal passion. The message is clear. There is no 'hard and fast' rule – if you'll pardon the pun.

Final myth: women want men who can keep it up all night.

Wrong. Women want men who can make love all night. Two very different concepts. Long sex does not necessarily mean long intercourse. In fact, for many, the thought of a long session of intercourse brings to mind the 'O' word – not orgasm, 'Ouch!'

All jokes aside, these male torments are growing to epidemic proportions with the increasing social emphasis on getting it up. Whilst women grieve about aging, this new obsession with *dickus erectus* is fast shaping up to be the 1990s male equivalent to the female beauty myth, and just as tragic.

I'm waiting for Calvin Klein to release a range of designer underpants that cater for those ten pound dumbbells. Then we'll all know we're in trouble.

NOT TONIGHT, JOSEPHINE

What has happened to male libidos? Have women's sex drives increased dramatically or have men just gone into a sudden decline en masse?

This is the question being asked around the world in reaction to the alarming statistics that show men are saying 'no' to sex in droves. No, non, nicht, are the sounds emanating from bedrooms across the globe, but contrary to the myth that it is wives and girlfriends who are turning a cold shoulder, it is the male of the species who seem to have gone off sex.

Theorists, therapists and researchers are at a loss to explain why women are knocking their doors down complaining about feeling frustrated. But having heard the cry from horny females myself over the past year – from girlfriends and even relatives – I decided to take a couple of months off to research the phenomenon of 'The Male Headache'.

What I discovered is this: Traditionally, women have had

their sexual peak whilst stuck at home, burdened with children and bogged down in domestica. The environmental 'curb' on women's sexuality generally suited the declining male.

Now more women are out in the workforce, exposed to attractive and stimulating people. Or they are freer in general as a result of child support, and such developments as HRT (hormone replacement therapy) which redresses many of the symptoms of menopause and aging. Thus women are able to fully enjoy and indulge in their libidinous urges. They are feeling sexier for longer, and looking better too.

Men are not widely being offered HRT with testosterone, even though it is becoming clear that men may also suffer some sort of andropause later in life. So medically speaking, older women may be biologically advantaged.

Away from hormones, and women are further spurred on by economic prosperity. In many cases women are now outstripping their husbands financially. A recent article in the reputable publication *Psychology Today* says we can no longer sweep female power under the cultural rug. 'Seven million American women earned more than their mates in 1993 and last year almost a quarter of all working wives out-earned their husbands.'

The fact is that women have changed profoundly as a result of economic independence, women's magazines, readily available child care and hormonal treatments.

The consequences are twofold. Women have become more demanding both in bed and out. This in turn is causing men to experience feelings of inadequacy, anger and resentment, fear, apprehension, confusion and stress which is directly impacting on their sex-lives, according to observers.

Psychologists quoted in *Psychology Today* say that many men are feeling 'castrated' or 'demoralised by changing roles'. Says one: 'I see in my practice an increase in the number of men who are reporting impotence and loss of sexual desire because they don't know how to behave any more.'

One of the most outspoken social commentators on this topic is Dr Sandra Pertot, author of *A Commonsense Guide to Sex* and an expert on sexual desire.

Dr Pertot, who has been a sex therapist since the '70s, told me her theories:

'Although historically it has been women who have had the headache, in at least half the couples I now see it is the men with the headache. The truth is that across the Western world men are avoiding sex in droves. I think it is because women have become too demanding.'

Dr Pertot feels there has been no decline in male libido, rather men are choosing to masturbate quietly in the privacy of their bathrooms. 'They can relax, retreat into their fantasies. They don't have to talk a woman into bed, perform and go through the criticism afterwards.

'In my clinical work I have found that the majority of men avoiding sex are still randy but they say sex with their partners is just not worth the effort.'

She says it is true that women are flocking to therapists and grizzling that their husbands don't want to have sex. But she says this is not a symptom of the problem. It is the cause of it. Whether a woman is working, or whether she has just fallen victim to the things she reads in women's magazines or sees at the movies, she is overwhelming men with her expectations. 'Women want too much,' she says.

'Men are being forced to compete with vibrators. One woman came to see me recently and criticised her man because he could only have sex for twenty minutes! She didn't realise twenty minutes is very good. Most men can have sex from two to ten minutes before there is some loss in erection, or ejaculation. Six minutes is quite normal.

'The average erection comes and goes – waxes and wanes. But women today aren't satisfied with this. They are taking more responsibility for their own sexual satisfaction but then they hold up their vibrators to their husbands and say, "Why can't you do this?" as if it is really his job.

'Nowadays women want orgasms with a cherry on top.'

Dr Pertot says she is disturbed by women regularly coming to see her complaining in front of their partners. 'This is creating a spotlight effect. The focus decreases male performance. And it is all wrong. What are we doing to our men? They feel like failures and inadequate because they can't last an hour.'

She says that many women have forgotten what sex is for. The biological imperative for the male is to ejaculate to impregnate the female. 'It is very hard for men to stop themselves ejaculating. Men are striving for physiological control all the time, whilst women strive to let go. We are putting unrealistic demands on men.'

Dr Debbie Then, sexpert and psychology PhD from Stanford University in the USA, who was recently in Australia doing research on strip-clubs and male–female relationships, took me off to a strip-club to watch the men ogle the female talent.

Whilst we were observing the cheering throng she told me that she agrees that more men are choosing alternatives to sleeping with their wives or partners.

'There has been a dramatic increase around the Western world in men seeing "professional girlfriends" as callgirls and prostitutes are now known, or frequenting lap-dancing and strip-clubs. Men are losing interest in making it with their wives. Professional girlfriends are even replacing mistresses and affairs in many instances.'

She agrees with Dr Pertot that women may be inadvertently intimidating men. 'When women have their own money and independence it changes their whole way of behaving. One of the most popular fantasies for men is the "conquering" fantasy, deflowering the virgin, the man in charge, sweeping the woman off her feet.

'When a woman becomes more confident and starts saying "move over there" or "I want it this way" it scares the shit out of men. They feel they are back under Mummy's control and this is not very sexual for most men.

'For men, sex has as much to do with power and control as it does with pleasure and orgasm. Many men can't have sex unless they feel in control. The increase in women instigating sex, and of women in the workforce, is stripping men of this control.'

She says that men are used to saying: 'I make money, I make the rules.' Now they are doing what women used to do. They are saying 'no' to sex to recoup the power and recover control in relationships where they feel they have lost their status. 'Turning you down means that they are calling the shots.'

She says the great irony in all of this is that most powerful women still want and get turned on by men who are more powerful and successful and wealthier than they are. The confusion is driving men crazy.

She says female sexual experience is also terrifying men and leading to performance anxiety. 'Before, only men were sexually experienced. Now men fear that a woman will judge him and find him incompetent or think that he's not doing it "right". With the stripper or "professional girlfriend" this is not the case. She is totally into him with no strings attached, no demands and no emotions. 'He doesn't have to perform,' she says as the buxom female playmates in the strip-club we are visiting pull off their scanty tops and perform around us.

But not all agree that women are impacting so strongly on men. Dr Michael Lowy of the Australian Centre for Sexual Health who I go to talk to for a male perspective suggests that the high rate of men presenting with sexual problems could simply be because there are so many impotency clinics springing up. This means that more men and their partners are now talking openly about, and dealing with, problems that have always existed.

Whatever the case, all therapists I talked to agree there is a problem that needs a solution. But they equally agree it will take time for the ripples caused by changing gender roles to iron out and for both sexes to find some sort of balance and equilibrium. In the meantime Dr Sandra Pertot has a word of advice for both men and women: 'Lighten up, for God's sake. Have some fun. It's only sex.'

GNOCCHI MAN

My husband's version of events goes something like this. There he was minding his own business, quietly kneading his own gnocchi in the Italian cooking course he was attending, when a woman started to come on to him.

Not overtly. Just in the subtle way that single women in cooking courses do. 'Do you want some help banging your gnocchis into shape?' she asked as he struggled with his mixture of flour and water.

'Ah, no,' he allegedly said trying to avoid her piercing gaze as flour went everywhere.

He gets a lot of piercing gazes from women, my husband. For one simple reason. He is very interested in women. He is the proverbial SNAG. He listens in to my conversations with my girlfriends, always offering an opinion. He runs off on Saturdays and books himself in to courses called 'Cooking with Garlic' or 'Latin Love Songs'. Last month he fair-dinkum did a course called 'A Guide to Tender, Loving, Intimate Communications'.

Not surprisingly, he attracts female patronage. Although he is indeed handsome and charming, I think it has more to do with the fact that he is usually the only man in the class.

Most men I know would rather be tortured with an electric cattle prod than attend a two-day seminar with fifty women bemoaning the fact that men don't listen to them – in fact, most men would actually see it as the same thing.

He does other warm and fuzzy things. Each morning before I stir, he takes our little girl down to the local park so she can play on the swings and slides under the watchful eye of other mothers.

There are always women on the phone who claim to have met my husband 'down at the sandpit' who ring to chat with him and to invite our baby to their kiddies' parties.

He is a pleasure to be in a relationship with, except that a lot of other women obviously agree.

I remember an episode of the TV show *Seinfeld* where one of the characters had 'Kavorca' – a mythical European word meaning 'the lure of the beast'. The lure of bad, sexually charismatic men on women.

Although I previously wrote that women are powerfully drawn to mad, bad men, I think my husband has another curse.

'Kavorci' – the lure of the gentle, sensitive man, who likes to cook, read poetry, take children to the park and do self-help courses that plum the depth of the inner man. An irresistible force that drives women out of their sandpits, and away from their gnocchis.

So, back to my husband's version of events. There he was, trying hard to ignore this woman in his Italian cooking course. Even though she was extremely attractive. Even though he admits: 'Her breasts were very pleasing to the eye.' (Sorry, girls. Even sensitive men notice.)

'You really need someone to show you how to squeeze those flour balls,' she said, leaving her own workbench and coming over to where he was making an unholy mess.

Having now studied intimate communication, he knew that he had to be very clear with this woman. 'Women are apt to see the world through their own romantic eyes. A female's yearning for love may lead her to misconstrue a hello for a *Hellllooooo*,' he told me on returning from his intimate bonding class the week before.

But before he blinked, his gnocchis were being pummelled skilfully into the workbench. She grabbed another lump of dough and glanced meaningfully into his face. 'You have to add more water to this so that it does not become too stiff,' she said, dribbling her water over his dough.

As he grew all flushed with male hormones she popped the question: 'So do you cook for yourself?'

And this is where men get themselves into trouble – even men who do communications courses. It's called male ego.

'Ummmm, I cook for myself and ... ummmm ... the other people in my house,' he said, leaving the door wide open enough for her continued attentions.

So the next thing, I am surfing the net and go to read my mail, and there are these recipes for vegetarian dishes and a rather florid description of things my husband might want to do with them.

All from the gnocchi lady who in my husband's version of events 'forced' his email address out of him as he 'struggled to rush home' (presumably to the 'other people' in the house) at the end of the course.

Kavorci. He certainly has it. It's hot and furious and dangerous stuff. To all the men who write in to me every week asking where all the women are, my husband would like to offer you this advice:

If you can tolerate hours of studying poetry, massage, self-help, communication, talking to whales or spending a few hours each week in the park with your neighbour's screaming kids, looking kind and sensitive, you will never have to worry about being lonely again. Although, on second thoughts, you may find being lonely a preferable option.

LITTLE LIES

When I was young I dated a man who behaved most oddly when I used to visit. After we'd done the deed, he'd get out a dust buster and start vacuuming the bed. He claimed to be allergic to hair.

It never occurred to me that there might be something a little odd in this behaviour. In fact, it wasn't until many months after we had broken up that I discovered that he was actually married to the woman he had claimed was 'just' his 'room-mate'.

When I confronted him on what I'd discovered he was unfazed, claiming that he had not lied to me. He just failed to tell me something that he considered 'irrelevant' at the time.

Likewise, he did not think his dalliance with me was something his wife needed to know about. 'It would only upset her,' he explained. 'It was for her sake I was so careful. Why cause her unnecessary pain?'

This story came to mind last week when a very funny list found its way onto my desk called: '101 Lies Men Tell Women' from a book of the same name by Dory Hollander. I laughed so much I nearly fell off my chair.

The list of porkies include: 'I'll call you'; 'I've never felt this way about anyone'; 'You're the only one I have sexual fantasies about'; 'My wife and I lead separate lives'; 'I've only slept with maybe ten women my entire life'; 'I haven't seen her since she and I broke up'; 'How could you think I'd be interested in her? She's your best friend!'

Some of my favourites include: 'I've never had any trouble keeping an erection before'; 'Your career is as important as mine'; 'I spend everything I earn on you and the kids'; 'No, I'm not having an affair'; 'Of course I'm listening to what you're saying.'

'Relax, she's just a friend'; 'Of course I'm not bored with you'; 'Come on in, and we'll just cuddle for a few minutes'; 'How many times do I have to tell you. I'm not having an affair!'

I found it amusing to note that most male lies were linked to sex and fidelity.

Seems men lie an average of five to fifteen times a week, according to a study done on male fibs that I reported on a couple of years ago. When I showed this figure to a number of men they were aghast, claiming that they never lied that much.

But they failed to take into account the 'white lies' they told to save people's feelings. Particularly 'women' people's feelings. 'I love that dress on you'; 'Of course you are beautiful'; 'You don't look fat at all'. They also generally forgot about 'grey lies' which are where a man will simply omit to tell you something he deems unnecessary to the situation or which may cause pain to someone – usually himself.

Whilst it is not exclusively male to fib, it seems it is extremely male to deny one is actually doing it. Take for instance the following vignette: Very few of the men I showed this to thought that the omission of detail was an outright 'black' lie.

A man is consistently late home from work. His wife confronts him asking him if he is having an affair with someone in the office. 'No,' he says, passionately. He is not having an affair with someone from the office. He does not furnish her with the information that he is having an affair with someone he met at a recent party.

'Well, he was being factual,' sniffed one male. 'And he would only hurt her and cause an argument if he told the truth.'

Our research has shown that not getting into trouble is the single most important motivating force in provoking men to tell lies. Faced with the prospect of an angry female face – indeed the face of mother – beaming down at them, or doing a sideward scuttle, the scuttle is overwhelmingly favoured.

Most men I talked to reckoned that 'honesty' following a lie, particularly if accompanied by tears of remorse, negated the original lie.

But the ones men seem to lie to most, are themselves. According to psychologists many men spend their lives denying their frailties, feelings and doubts in order to cope. 'I'm okay' is the most common male fib.

The million-dollar question is: Do men lie more than women or just differently?

Men are certainly more creative at the art. Take the scenario of scratch marks on the back. Here are three real-life excuses offered to women by men I know: One said he had rolled onto the cat in bed. One said he was raking the garden without a shirt on and was scratched by a low-hanging tree. But the final one is the best:

He said he scratched himself because he'd been bitten by a mosquito. He failed to see that his arms would have had to have been ten foot long to have created those marks – I guess about as long as the tall tales so many men tell us long, long suffering women.

LAPPING IT UP

The room is so filled with smoke you feel like you are about to be gobbled up. All around the walls are photos of naked female bodies. There is a surreal and almost eerie feeling to The Governor's Pleasure – a 'lingerie' restaurant in the heart of Sydney.

With all the controversy that surrounded the latest spate of strip-tease movies and the raging world-wide resurgence of the art of stripping and lap-dancing, I have decided to take a girl-friend along to see what goes on in one of these joints.

I am told that there will be a three-course meal served. Between each course the waitresses who are walking around in their underwear, will strip down to bare essentials.

I am also informed that women like me rarely frequent the place despite its reputation as a more 'up-market' haunt situated in the centre of town to attract the corporate market. Apparently women feel 'uncomfortable'.

Despite the smoke, it is not hard to make out the waitresses. Clad in lacy bras that lift their bosoms to chin height, garter belts, G-strings, black stockings and lots of cascading hair, they lean provocatively over the customers and rub their tushes closer than most regular waitresses would ever dare.

Once my eyes have acclimatised to this extraordinary vision, I begin noticing the clientele. Blokes in loud shirts, with loud voices smoking and drinking vast quantities of alcohol. Slowly, I begin to notice that a room full of eyes are trained on my blonde girlfriend and I.

Trained and strained. Some are almost boggling out of their heads. It's like a scene from some spooky movie where the heroine suddenly realises that the walls are moving, crawling with something deadly. I realise that we are not journalists, mothers or people – merely women. Women with slightly more clothes on than the other 'creatures of pleasure' swanning around the room.

In here it isn't just clothing that is stripped away for females – it is the veneer of civilisation we pretend exists. In here men are at their most primordial and I am just a female genital with some bits and pieces attached to make movement possible.

'Aaahh!' a waitress screams, complaining she has been bitten on the bum. 'Animal,' she curses showing us the bruise. 'They think because we're in our underwear they can do anything to us.'

Suddenly the lights go down, and eyes move away from us to the stage. One of the waitresses has started dancing – bumping and grinding on a long, gold pole.

She moves over to a table and asks one of the men to take off her top. He is trembling so much he can't unfasten her bra. 'C'arn . . . you virgin,' someone yells as the men wait in breathless anticipation and palpable frustration. As if seeing this breast, at this moment in time, is the most consuming, desperate need of their entire existence.

The clip unfastens. A loud sigh is heard across the room. A

wave of pleasure and relief ... 'Aaaaaah', they moan together. 'Oooooh'.

The stripper mounts the stage and again dances. A few wild cheers are heard but mainly there is a captivated silence. The men are awestruck. One man has been straining so hard to see, he has fallen out of his chair. Another is tilted vertically across the table to get a better view. The girl rubs oil into herself. The tension is rising. You can feel the heat, almost smell the oozing testosterone. It is like nothing I have ever felt before.

If you were alone you would be mauled alive. These are lions and the tamer has them transfixed, but for how long?

Then it happens. The G-string comes off. She is naked, and shiny and moving around in mesmerising rhythm.

I look around the room. The eyes are focused in worship. It is pure love. The yearning so strong, the emotions so high, I think some men are about to cry. It is pure adoration. It is religion. These men are in a trance. And then it dawns on me. I see the truth.

This woman, all women – we have power. And the power we wield is awesome and frightening. At this moment these men are slaves, docile in their worship. They would do anything: cross deserts, dive into shark-infested waters, for one small grope of that breast. For one touch of that sacred spot from whence they came.

'The power of the muff' one of my boyfriends used to call it. 'It can lead men to war. No man can resist it. Women don't understand how truly powerful they are.'

The light comes on, and as my girlfriend and I get up to leave, every eye is again on us, longingly, lustfully.

And I wonder what it is about this particular type of power – the power of female sexuality – that has disturbed feminists so greatly, that they want to lock it up and denounce it. For this short moment, I strut proudly out of that restaurant, wielding the power of my sexuality with a deep, gleeful, guilty joy.

ALL NIGHT LONG

I've got to be honest here. I'm not the kind of babe that goes in for hours and hours of passion. For me sex is like eating chocolate. I make myself put the block down whilst I'm still wanting, so I can look forward to it the next time around.

There is nothing worse than scoffing down the entire family-sized block then feeling bad, overindulged, guilty, and ready to throw up.

So a recent book that crossed my path *How to Make Love All Night*, by American sex therapist Barbara Keesling – about how men can become multi-orgasmic and keep going all night – really had me wondering.

The premise of course its that everybody wants to make love all night. Everyone wants to just do it over and over again for hours and hours like a sexual Olympics marathon: '*And they're going for Gold. Yes! Seventeen hours, ladies and gentlemen. A world record! What a wonderful moment for Australia!*'

Apparently the book sold very well overseas, which has me stumped. I once did it all night when I was younger. Hours of unbridled passion until the dawn broke, burning lust, and then more burning lust. Burning being the operative word.

'Oouch!' was all I could say for the next week as I limped around Bali beach struggling to come to terms with the anatomical damage I had done to my person.

Because the sad truth is that no matter how happy and smirky Barbara Keesling looks on the dustjacket of the book, there is only so much passion a body can tolerate. Particularly female bodies that come with bladders inside.

Worse news is that when I rang a bookshop to find out the details of the book, I was told there is another book out on how to make love for several days straight. Non-stop. Bop until you drop (dead that is).

I suppose that if one's body made love all night, every night, one's body would eventually accommodate the rigours of sex, much the same way my fingertips learned to cope with my rampant guitar strumming by growing calluses.

But it begs the next question: Who has the time and energy to make love all night, every night, to get one's body acclimatised? Who even has the time to make love?

And it's all very well to write a book that helps men get more control over their bods so they can orgasm again and again. But do men really want multiple orgasms? Most of the men I have known tell me the best part of sex for them is the sleep afterwards.

Whilst women presumably like to bask in the afterglow, men tend to fall into a deep, relaxed state called 'Post-Coital Somnambulance'. In the dictionary this is described as a 'comatose-state' resembling zombiism, 'a hypnotic trance' and a 'state of sleepwalk'.

Men love this deep, sleep-like relaxation. It's like a beer at the end of a game of footy or tennis. It's the 'Aaaaahhh' of intimacy. They make weird snoring noises and any further conversation or act of love is peacefully carried out with their eyes closed.

Now they are being told by books and women's magazines that they can have sex all night and maybe that they *should* be having sex all night – because that's what we multi-orgasmic, modern femmes want.

Well the truth of the matter is that women may indeed have

the potential for endless bliss. But we're all so busy feeding children, running busy careers and households and exercising to stay beautiful and beat the aging process – in short being Superwoman – that we're more likely to be narcoleptic than orgasmic. [Narcolepsy: 'Sudden and uncontrollable episodes of deep sleep'.]

Most women I know can't even look at a bed without falling asleep. In fact, I think that Barbara Keesling has grossly underestimated the intoxicating and irresistible lure of the sandman.

Anyway, for those who desperately do want to know the secret of making love all night, it is all in the muscles.

It is possible, according to the sexperts, for men to climax or have some sort of peak sexual experience, without ejaculating. Much of the current wisdom in this area has come from Eastern lovemaking traditions.

Keesling says that the way for the average man to gain control of his sexual responses is to do PC muscle exercises. Any man whose wife has had a baby will know about the old PCs. Women exercise them prenatally to help control labour, and to stop incontinence and improve orgasm after labour.

Men have the same muscles and by exercising them for substantial periods of time every day, can apparently gain control over ejaculation and have multiple orgasms without the release of sperm. An excellent local book on this is *Loving Longer, Loving Stronger* by Kundan Misra [Gambol Books].

My poor, long-suffering husband has been practising these exercises stoically for the past two weeks so I could truthfully report to you on whether he became multi-orgasmic or not.

But sadly there has been a problem. He has put so much time and energy into exercising his PC muscles he is too exhausted to be 'tested out'. I've turned him into a multi-orgasmic narcoleptic.

THE MALE PEACOCK

Anyone a bit stumped by Paul Hogan's recent transformation from a rugged, bronzed Aussie with craggy good looks, to a somewhat smoother-faced dude who looks as if an iron has been run under his eyes, be consoled. Our very own Paul is not the only bloke to have seemingly tampered with what nature gave him in recent times.

Latest statistics from the Academy of Cosmetic Surgery show that men now account for over 25 per cent of facelifts and plastic surgery patients in America, with doctors agreeing that the trend is fast catching on here.

One of the reasons for the trend is the fact that the workforce is getting younger by the minute, and now with downsizing and outsourcing, many men feel enormous pressure to look younger than their years to remain employable.

But the other reason is the increasingly common phenomenon of overt male vanity. It is a widely held myth that it is the female of the species who preens and is obsessed with physical beauty.

Not so. Just as it has always been the male peacock who has flashed his coloured, throbbing bits during the mating dance, so too were the men of ancient Greece the ones who were consumed by the notion of aesthetic beauty. Now, over the past decade, there has been a dramatic resurgence in cosmetic alterations that help men appear more sexually potent.

According to a friend of mine who lives in Los Angeles there is a significant hike in men having 'ball-tucks' (scrotum tightening operations) to make their testicles look firmer and more inviting. I have written recently about penis extension operations that are thriving around the world for purposes of vanity rather than performance. Men are being injected with liposuctioned fat in the lower regions as well as using dumbbells to extend their members.

As for the illusion of grandeur, an amusing trend amongst gay males is now spreading to the straight community. This is where the male, before going out on the prowl, gets a large stone and rubs a huge white area into the crotch of his jeans to create the appearance of fulsome apparatus. At its most extreme, this also includes sewing a shoulder-pad into the crotch.

For those in disbelief, I have had a personal experience with shoulder-pads. One well-built and handsome fellow I dated for a while always insisted on making love with his pyjama top on. I never objected because I accept that people have strange sexual habits. But he also always wore a T-shirt when sunbathing — in the days before skin cancer was an issue.

One day I dropped in unexpectedly whilst he was in the shower and noticed that his shirts, T-shirts, jackets and even pyjama tops all had shoulder-pads sewn in so it would always look as if he had a hunky body.

I have known many men who have sported beards. Often when you look at their childhood or teenage photos, you'll notice a not entirely flattering chin structure.

I have dated at least two men who have used beauty creams before bed and one who, when his eyes got red from contact lenses or after a few too many drinks, would actually draw a faint brown line inside his eye and around it, with my eyeliner.

When I commented on a male friend's hair colour recently, implying that the grey bits were a bit aging, he promptly went and got it dyed.

The fact is that there is no shame in male vanity. And it

should become more socially acceptable. Men do age, and why shouldn't they also try to make the most of what nature gave them?

It is folly for men to continually berate women for not sporting the body beautiful whilst they allow themselves to bloat and sag and look bad. A recent report on male obesity in this country was most alarming, revealing that a huge percentage of Aussie men are overweight and slobby. Guys wouldn't tolerate it from women.

Like women, aging men have all sorts of traits that make them unattractive. When men age their ears grow bigger and also become hairier. Older men often grow breasts, a funny yet sad phenomenon recently dealt with on the TV show *Seinfeld* where the characters were trying to design a bra for older men to help with this very embarrassing and prevalent problem.

It is common when you live with a man to find him with your tweezers up his nose, plucking out the sprouts of hair or trimming them.

And yet all this has to be done in stealth. Aussie men find it humiliating or a sign of weakness to buy their own tweezers, face creams, or hair conditioners, quite unlike Italian and European men who demand product ranges to adorn themselves and improve their innate beauty.

I am all for male vanity, as long as men don't take it too far. And I think most women would agree that it will be a great day when we no longer have to hide the tweezers and nail scissors for fear of where they may end up.

BASTARDS

There's been a lot of bleating and complaining by women recently behind boardroom doors, and over executive lunches, that men have become a little too New Age. Too sensitive. 'A bit like emotional jellyfish,' one girlfriend complained. 'Geldings,' grumbled another.

In fact, women have been moaning to me that the whole experiment into New Age maleness has been a bit like a cake gone wrong. We wanted a dash of kindness and consideration and a smidgen of sweetness thrown into the ingredients to create a sort of New Age Neanderthal. A testosterone-riddled male who would drag you by the hair into his cave and ravish you, then make you a cappuccino afterwards and discuss 'the relationship'.

But girls are now whispering to each other in the corridors of power that maybe someone misunderstood the recipe and poured too much syrup into the cake, leaving us with a sticky, spongy thing that won't rise to the occasion.

Well, girls, you can relax and stop fretting. If a new survey just out of the United States is anything to go by most men haven't changed all that much, after all.

Although some men have gone a bit marshmallowy, prancing about on bonding weekends, weeping and dangling from trees in search of their manhood, the fact is that when it comes to bedroom manners and sexual etiquette most men are still dishing out the same old unreconstructed behaviour they are infamous for.

American Dialogue, a New York City research firm that interviewed 1000 men across the country aged between eighteen and thirty-four for *Mademoiselle* magazine, put the question: 'You've been dating a fantastic woman and you know tonight is "the night". You also just heard that you are to be transferred indefinitely to your company's office in Australia. When do you break the news to her?'

Almost half of the males interviewed said they would wait till after they had sex with the poor woman before letting her in on the secret.

When asked in a multiple-choice question what a man was able to do with another woman without feeling like a cheat: 64 per cent said they could flirt comfortably, 42 per cent could take another woman to dinner, 22 per cent could happily kiss another woman, 13 per cent could do everything but have intercourse whilst at least 7 per cent could happily have a drunken one-night stand without feeling bad.

When asked the question, 'You just slept with a woman for the first time at your place. She'd like to stay over but you want her to leave', 42 per cent would let her stay. But the majority said they would either tell her flatly to go or make up some excuse to get rid of her. Meanwhile the average time men thought they should continue cuddling a woman after sex was twenty minutes, and when it came to oral sex 64 per cent thought between one to twenty minutes was 'a good faith effort' *regardless* of the outcome.

Almost half of men interviewed said that the only mistake Hugh Grant made was getting caught, with well over a quarter of men admitting to having visited a prostitute.

How long would a man wait before asking a woman's girl-friend on a date after a breakup? Most Sensitive New Age Guys would hit on the best friend within a few weeks to a few months, with only 28 per cent finding this off limits. As for the male competitive spirit – the majority of men would not stop trying to seduce a woman just because they saw a wedding ring on her finger.

Less than half of the men would tell a woman he had herpes well before sexual contact (if he intended wearing a condom) while an alarming 55 per cent of men would not wear a condom with their partner after having an unsafe fling in case she became suspicious.

Nearly half of the men interviewed felt entitled to pressure a woman from lightly to heavily for sex after they had paid for four consecutive dates, while a significant 43 per cent of men would stop seeing a woman if she had not 'delivered' by the fifth date regardless of who was footing the bill.

Over 60 per cent of men had encouraged a woman to drink in order to increase his chances of having sex whilst over two-thirds of men don't believe a man is obliged to see a woman again after having sex with her, if he's lost interest.

Another recent survey on sex and pornography found that a quarter of the male population read *Playboy* with many men admitting they read 'girlie' magazines because they could 'interact with an attractive woman without having to deal with a troublesome personality'.

So it seems the Sisterhood is grieving the loss of testosterone in the male species prematurely. Or could it be that we've stopped trying to rid the world of bad male behaviour because the cure is far worse than the disease?

BOYS AND THEIR THINGS

Twice a year, when the moon is full and the mood is right, the men at one of Sydney's leading stockbroking firms throw away their grey business suits and partake in a very secret, very special ritual. It is a ritual much like those found in pagan times – a rite of manhood, a rite of sexual potency and prowess.

On these sacred days the partners of the firm and some of the senior analysts and dealers take their throbbing red and black Porsches, their sports cars and Mercs or European hot rods they have had brought in specially for the occasion, to a well-known race track in Sydney, hire the leading racing experts and pay for the track to be theirs for the afternoon.

And then, like ancient warriors, these fellows – who in real life drive very slowly so they can concentrate on their mobile telephone discussions – become untamed beasts who drive their machines round and round and round in ferocious circles, competing to see which man emerges as the meanest, fastest most macho driver, with the hottest, fastest, most powerful machine.

For weeks beforehand the boys hold special meetings about the day which is fast approaching. As the event grows closer, so do the boys at the firm. A source tells me they start nestling together in groups or couples. Boasting and cooing about their machines as if they were describing the most passionate love of their life. Men who never talked together for any length of time are suddenly locked in intense dialogue about their driving technique, fast cars they have driven, horrific and near fatal accidents they have been involved in.

The older, more experienced partners take one of the younger dealers aside and with arm on shoulder and great poignancy and tenderness they whisper profound wisdom like: 'Remember to cut the corners finely', or 'Just open the throttle and go'.

Oh, boys with their toys. Men of the '90s may be learning to be deep and sensitive. They may wash dishes and cook exquisite meals for their executive wives. They may be caring and sharing to a degree. But deep down they are still more comfortable with *things* than feelings, still need hard objects or events to communicate with and through.

Talking shop, or sport, is still easier than ripping into the gut. Racing cars and competing is an easier testimony to success and selfhood than sharing information about your emotional life or inner self. Men still don't know how to let go of their *things*, not when they are with women and certainly not when they are together.

I have noticed that when out with males, even the more communicative types, very early in the evening a thing will be brought out to impress me or distract me. A phallic symbol. A throbbing new red car. A house with a harbour view which then becomes the focus of conversation for the rest of the night.

Sensitive men will show you the painting they have just acquired: an antique copy of some famous novel they got at auction, the expensive cast-iron French cooking pots that they had imported from Paris for their dinner parties.

If men haven't got their *thing* on them, they will describe it to you in vivid, loving detail: the horses they have sitting up at some farm, the valuable carving they dragged back from a trek in India. Their conquest.

How they handle the *thing* is very important. Control over the *thing* is paramount because it denotes performance and winning. So they'll describe mastery over their yacht, horse, tennis racquet or cooking pots with great verve like the peacocks from the stockbroking firm bragging about their ability to drive round in circles, fast.

Time and time again men cling onto their *thing* while I struggle to lead conversation away from the *thing* into a more esoteric or intimate zone. But getting a man to let go of his *thing* is not easy. He'll wince and keep coming back to it. Clutching onto it as if it is a life raft that will help him stay afloat in the messy emotional chaos which is feelings, intimacy and women.

In my dating days I had to sit in the antique car of a male admirer as he drove it up and down the main drag of some outer suburb. I watched him fondling the gearstick with great pride. He kept turning to me and grinning. Later at home he made me help him polish the front of the machine.

When I felt sure he had made his statement and was feeling secure around his self-image, I tried to find out how he was feeling since his girlfriend abandoned him and how he'd been coping emotionally. He promptly opened the lid of his car to demonstrate his knowledge of the little wires around the engine.

Three weeks of dating this man and I knew more about his gearbox than his heart.

A divorcee I met a few years ago had lots of boys toys, *things* and gadgets around his home and he kept pressing buttons so his house would do tricks for me. As we spoke, drapes kept opening and shutting, music went on and off from speakers high above the room, a large video screen was touch-activated.

When I tried to broach the delicate subject of his separation he pressed some button and said: 'I bet you can't guess what that noise is,' as the bubbles from a jacuzzi started to froth and foam in a distant room.

Things. Things. Barriers and more barriers. By the end of the evening I was exhausted. If women find it so difficult to develop intimacy with a man, if extracting emotional information feels like pulling teeth, then what hope have men got together?

I guess anyone wandering down to the Sydney racecourse to watch macho stockbrokers doing wheelies, and playing with their *things* together, will find the answer to that question.

HEROES

As I have said, my husband is a Sensitive New Age Guy. He cooks, washes dishes, reads me poetry and performs lots of other touchy-feely type activities. But the minute an adventure film comes on the telly he is transformed into El Macho Supremo. He is Batman, he is Robin Hood, throwing himself about the apartment in commercial breaks with a puffed-out chest, speaking with a deeper voice about the time he held an Uzi gun, rode a horse or got stuck up a tree.

He may, for a while after the movie, do manly type things like lift me in his arms for no apparent reason and toss me in the air. Or he will prance around the flat nominating things that need hammering and sawing, and asserting he will fix them in a 'Trust-me-I'm-a-man' sort of voice.

Then, ultimately frustrated that there is no damsel to save, no maiden to impress and woo into the matrimonial bed, no arrow to shoot, no sword to wield – that the most heroic thing he can do is to help me unscrew the child-proof painkiller bottle lid – he will return to himself.

Like most boys he grew up with a host of TV and comic book idols: Superman (able to leap tall buildings in a single bound), Zorro, Mighty Mouse. And like most boys he is coming to a time in his life when he is realising he may never be *Star Trek's* Captain James Kirk – boldly going where no man has ever gone before, seeking out new galaxies … which is where my story begins.

I am of the belief that most men don't suffer a mid-life crisis. It is in fact a *Captain Kirk Crisis*. It is the culmination of years of disappointment and frustration at never having saved a damsel, bedded a princess, ridden a horse into the sunset or saved a galaxy.

Which is why I took no notice of a tale my darling husband told me on my return from overseas.

He: 'While you were away this whole building nearly burned down. There were flames everywhere. The sky was burning red.' Then, thrusting out his chest. 'I saved everyone's life . . . I single-handedly saved the building.'

Me: 'Wonderful, dear. You'll tell me about it later. Are there any urgent bills to attend?'

He: 'I must tell you this story.'

I looked at his face. The need to be Superman was intense. So I sat quietly on the couch while he enacted the scenario. Flames were licking the back of the building from a shed that was on fire below. Because of the density of trees in the area and the raging winds, the flames would surely engulf the surrounding houses.

The firemen couldn't get to the flames because of obscured access. While they scurried about working out how to douse the soaring flames, my husband had a brilliant idea.

At this stage he dragged me to the window to view the charred remains of trees and the blackened facade of my building. I saw nothing but greenery and the usual array of flowers so I figured we were looking at an exaggeration somewhere in the vicinity of a million to one. That my darling had probably spotted a smouldering barbecue someone had forgotten to douse. But I forced an impressed look onto my female face.

He had the idea to drag the fire hose from our building through the window of a nearby apartment. While panic and pandemonium reigned below and the flames climbed higher into the night, he bravely turned on the hose. The water gushed onto the fire. The flames died. He saved hundreds of lives and millions of dollars of property single-handedly. The fire department and those standing below clapped and cheered him.

Unfortunately, it was dark, he said, so no-one actually saw his face. No-one actually knows the hero is him. He is an unsung hero but a hero nonetheless.

'Mmmmmm …' I said. 'Wonderful, darling. Wonderful.' Then I went off to attend to urgent letters leaving my unsung hero to face his *Captain Kirk Crisis alone*.

Many months went by. But recently, as fate would have it, he and I were asked to attend a meeting of the neighbourhood to discuss a building proposal for our area. One neighbour said he objected to the new building which would be built in the park below our apartment block, on the grounds that it was a fire hazard.

'Remember that fire a few months ago? The whole park nearly went up in smoke, and us along with it,' he said.

'One man saved all our lives. He dangled bravely from that window up there. He put out the flames single-handedly. He is a hero. He deserves a bravery medal from the fire department. But no-one knows who he is.'

'It was that man!!' said one fellow, pointing to my husband. 'I saw him from my flat over there.'

My darling was glowing. 'Yes,' he said, stepping forward, his voice deepening again, 'it was me.'

Ten big men ran over and threw their arms around him. Twenty women thanked him for saving their families. The meeting was alive with praise.

'You could have died, dangling out of that window!' one woman said loudly.

'Yes,' said my darling with his head held high. 'I could have been killed … easily.'

And I could see from the expression on his face and the way he was standing that this was the most precious, beautiful, fulfilling and perfect moment of his entire life.

DREAMING OF PAMMY

New American research has shown that every time a woman reads a glossy magazine, her adrenalin drops and she goes into a slight depression because of the beautiful bodies she sees. I don't know why. It is an undeniable, indisputable and awesomely strange fact: the more beautiful my single girlfriends, the less luck they seem to have getting men into bed.

I have taken strong note of this social phenomenon over the years, beginning my research in my wild single days.

We would go out for evenings, my single girlfriends and I, all dressed to kill, high-heeled, come-love-me shoes and lipstick painted on our lips having dieted for months to squeeze into our pencil-tight skirts so we could resemble the babes we saw in glossy magazines. We were a true bevy of beauties, but although men would circle us in nightclubs giving us the greasy eyeball, very few ever moved in for the kill.

But there was one girl in our clan who got lucky wherever we went, even if we were out drinking coffee.

Whilst we dieted ourselves into near oblivion, torturing our bodies till we looked like boys in drag, this voluptuous creature ate – with gusto and verve – every morsel on her plate. And whilst she certainly would not have made it through an audition of *Baywatch*, amazingly, astoundingly, unbelievably, that woman had more sex than the six of us put together. Men simply adored her, drawn inexplicably to her abundant appetites, her infectious laughter and her happy demeanour.

Over the years I saw the situation recur. Whilst many of the beautiful women I knew, full of diet pills and high expectations, were whining about the lack of sex, or trouble they had with partners during sex – premmie ejaculators and the like – the simpler, plainer women I knew were very, very lucky in love.

So what does one make of this phenomenon? Having thought about it over the decades, I conclude that although we are all bombarded to the point of exhaustion with images of the blonde bimbette and the honey-coloured love child on TV commercials, in shows like *Baywatch* and in glossy magazines, which leave us feeling inadequate, this is not an image men want of us – not in reality, that is.

Men may fantasise about Pamela Anderson with her gorgeous boobs and long blonde hair but how many could actually feel, in their deepest hearts, that they could sustain an erection long enough and big enough to satisfy the sex goddess?

It would seem from talking to all the men I know that most of them have an issue with potency. They are terrified to death they won't perform. How much more terrifying to have to lie down with a perfectly shaped babe who is no doubt expecting a magnificent performance? I think the reality is that most men would probably prefer to have a tooth extracted or a toenail torn off than to have to go through the humiliating agony of bedding an Elle.

My men friends tell me that when they are in the arms of a flawed creature, they can relax. They can stop tensing the muscles in their abdomens and let their tummies fall loose. They can hoist themselves up in a host of wonderful and highly unflattering positions and they don't even have to apologise if they pull a muscle in their backs or, God forbid, fail to raise the dead. Hey, everyone in this bed is only human, right? (Well, one hopes.)

There is nothing hornier in the world than feeling relaxed and comfortable with your partner, so intimate you can let go totally. Let's face it, the sex act, with the light on and without Vaseline on the camera lens, ain't very flattering to either party.

Despite what women might think, I have found from personal experience that most men are truly oblivious of cellulite during the act. If anything, men like a bit of 'schmaltz' on the bum or hips in sex: something extra to grab onto in those slippery moments like those rubber bathmats at the foot of a shower. An anchor of love, so to speak, to stop them rolling about too much or toppling off.

And anyway most men are not thinking about your thighs because they are too busy worrying about whether or not they are doing an okay job at it, poor bastards.

I'm not saying that men don't fantasise about Pamela Anderson whilst lying down with normal women. God only knows I would if I were a bloke. There is nothing wrong with a bit of aesthetic yearning and lust in the privacy of one's head. I know, too, from research I have done, that one of the favourite male fantasies is the deflowering or 'conquering' fantasy in which the Pammy creature is all breathless and vulnerable and waiting for love.

In reality, of course, the Pammy creature has expectations and needs that terrify the average bloke half to death. Hence life experience has taught me that deep down where it counts, men are contented with their womenfolk just the way we are. In the privacy of their own bedrooms, they are voting with their bodies to allow us our curved bellies from child-bearing, our stretch-marks and the laugh and character lines on our faces. Otherwise none of us would be getting laid, right?

But out in public, it seems that men are as much victims of

the same sad beauty myth that forces women to feel miserable every time they read a glossy magazine, and our teenaged daughters to become anorexic.

They are almost forced to sport a drop-dead gorgeous, perfect specimen on their arm to impress their mates. Worse, men have to say things to each other each day like, 'God, I'd like to give 'er one,' while pointing to some hapless female – an odd bonding ritual, equivalent to women saying to each other 'Hello, how are you?'

We should change the rules and follow the European example where men overtly and publicly admire women at all stages and ages of life. Europeans celebrate the fecundity of the female form in all its Rubenesque loveliness. It's time our men found the courage and compassion to start speaking the truth – for all our sakes.

MALE MASSAGE

We are standing in a dimly lit room, my husband and I, waiting for an appointment with a man called Chester Mainard. My husband looks like a cat about to be handed over to the vet. I take his hand to give him reassurance that he is doing the right thing. He pulls away, muttering angrily to himself about being 'forced' into this.

All weekend we have been fighting about this meeting. Mainard is an internationally renowned sex educator, visiting Australia to teach men about their sexuality.

When I find out the maestro of male sexuality is in town I suggest that my husband go to a workshop or to a private session so I can report his experiences. He gingerly agrees to do a one-on-one session with Mainard, then spends the next two days grizzling about it.

'What's he going to teach me that I don't already know?' he protests. I explain that from interviews I have been conducting with sex educators and male health experts across Australia, it is widely believed that men are very uneducated about the workings of their anatomies – particularly their genitals.

Mainard is a world expert in male private parts and their various functions. He can help men experience stronger orgasms, even multiple orgasms, I explain. He can teach men how to orgasm but not ejaculate. He is an expert on nerve endings in the lower regions of a man's body and can help increase pleasure.

My husband is sweating. Like most men, he has been conditioned since he was a boy to abstain from discussing his privates or even admitting he has any. Whereas women sit on the telephone endlessly bemoaning the various complaints of their lower regions, or discussing the latest *Cosmo* article on how to have simultaneous, multiple G spot orgasms, most men don't know the difference between their prostate and their perineum.

'What's he going to do to me?' my husband asks, wincing.

He works through deep relaxation and massage. 'Massage?' my husband yells. 'Massage?' and with that he is out the door.

This is not an uncommon reaction from men, Mainard assures me over the phone when I ring to explain the difficulty I am having locating my husband.

'Many of the men who come to see me are sent by nagging wives or girlfriends who want to improve their sex-lives by helping men get into their own bodies.

'It is a myth that most men are sexual beings. Men are not taught to be sexual in a way that allows them to enjoy their bodies, experience a deeper pleasure in an erotic, sensuous way.

Many men are still very much into performing in bed rather than sensing and feeling.'

US-born Mainard is a somatic psychotherapist and certified body worker with a Masters of Science in education. For fourteen years he instructed medical students at the University of Wisconsin in the art and science of male pelvic exams, and the physiology of the rectum. Mainard, like his mentor Joseph Kramer who pioneered the now-famous Body Electric School of body awareness in California, is one of a new band of male liberators who tour the world giving lectures and running workshops about the male body and its potential for pleasure.

According to Mainard and many of his peers, this is the next step in the so-called men's movement. To get men out of their heads, and into their bodies. 'Into their physical selves,' he says. 'The first stage was getting men to admit to their feelings but now they've got to learn how to feel those feelings, particularly in relation to sexuality.'

He says when he first started talking about these things, very few men were listening. Now his business is so popular all over the world – amongst gay and straight men – he is run off his feet. 'Just check out my frequent flyer points,' he laughs.

The sudden explosion of interest in male sexuality in Australia is very much in keeping with the new world trend. Several books keep hitting the shelves with men yearning for information about their health, their sexuality and their bodies.

The men are yearning for the information that women have been getting for years through books like *The Female Eunuch* and through magazines. They are ready for what book publishers describe as 'the common-sense side of the male movement'. Research in the publishing industry has shown that the market is ripe for picking.

Meanwhile Dr Michael Lowy from the Sydney Centre for Men's Health at St Luke's hospital in Sydney says that the sudden plethora of clinics for impotence or sexual problems indicates that men are finally prepared to be educated on the state of their bodies. 'They are beginning to feel safe.'

Gary Dowsett, lecturer in sociology at Macquarie University, agrees. 'You only have to look in the papers at all the ads for sexual clinics for men to see evidence of real change.'

He says that although talking about erection problems is a long way from developing the deeper erotic skills Chester Mainard teaches, it is the first step towards men becoming informed and thus sexually whole.

'There is a definite changing consciousness out there about being a man. Images in the media have started to portray the male body as erotic and sensuous. Being objectified as sexual creatures has caused a crisis for many men who have had to change the way they see themselves. It is no longer good enough to be desiring, men now have to be desirable too,' he says.

'As a result men are beginning to do something. It could be a workshop, or going to the gymnasium to improve their bodies, or visiting a clinic for a penis implant. But men are recognising that they need to be a sexual people too.'

It is strange to hear repeatedly that men are not sexual beings given that the world has always viewed the male as the more sexual of the species.

Norman Dean Radican who among other things is men's health educator at the Royal North Shore Hospital in Sydney says: 'Men have sex but they don't see themselves as being sexual. Men don't masturbate to give themselves pleasure, but to get off. How many men take the time for pleasure? It would never enter their heads to light a candle, put on some music and get into the other parts of their body.'

Meanwhile authors of *Sexual Secrets for Men*, Kerry and Diane Riley say that men are so busy trying to please women, they forget to please themselves. 'It's gone from one extreme to the other. Things have got to be brought back into balance.

'Women have gone through an incredible transformation in sexual awareness and men are scared they can't meet everything that is required. Historically sex for men has been simple – move until there is an explosion of energy. Now women are inundated with information and they want to be satisfied on many different levels. Men's pleasure is often determined by how well their women are feeling. Sex is more than ever a performance issue.'

Kerry Riley says: 'Men have never been taught to explore their own sexuality – their own ecstasy – sex is defined in narrow terms of orgasm and intercourse.' He says most men know little about areas such as the 'million dollar spot' which when pressed stops men ejaculating during orgasm. They don't know about all the nerve endings in and around their genitals, and around the prostate region. He says the book is aimed at educating people about the sexual ecstasy men are capable of.

So here we stand, my husband and I, waiting to see how Mainard puts his theories into practice and to see if sexual ecstasy is on the agenda.

We are now in a terrace in Sydney's Paddington where one of Mainard's protégés, masseur and sex educator Andre Dussart, carries on the work while Mainard is travelling.

Out of a shadowy corner Mainard appears. He is gentle and modest in disposition. I see my husband relax. But as Mainard leads him to a massage table and asks him to undress, he again peers at me like a trapped animal. I am certain he's about to bite Chester's hand and run away. Instead he slips off his clothes and lies naked on the table.

'What are your fears?' Chester asks gently. My husband admits he is fearful of being touched by another man. He is fearful of the homosexual overtones of the work. He is fearful of losing control. I know, that like many other men, he is fearful of feeling.

'You will control how far we go, how we will work,' Chester reassures him, kindly. 'Close your eyes. This is not about who is giving you the massage. It is not about whether your teacher is male or female, straight or gay. This work is about unlocking the flow of energy inside you. I am here to help you explore yourself.'

As he runs his hands over my husband's back, he gently explains that tension from the anger and frustration of living, are too often pushed deep inside of men with an emotional coffee plunger. As the emotions are suppressed, sexual energy is often pushed down with it.

Between sentences, Mainard breathes deeply, indicating my husband should follow. The emphasis is on the in-breath like sucking in a drink through a straw. I recognise the breath to be one used in Tantric ritual to help raise energy. In many circles it is known as the re-birth breath because people are known to go into strange, primal regressive states after such sessions.

Mainard says he uses the breath to help men deal with their issues before bringing them into focus with their sexuality.

I watch my husband relax into a euphoric state as the breathing quickens in tempo. Mainard then asks me to leave the room. This is men's stuff. Men's business. I sit reading in another room without concentrating.

An eternity later, my husband emerges. He looks serene. He stares out of the window in a trance. 'How was it?' I ask. 'Incredible,' he says but will not elaborate for days. When he finally speaks he talks of an odd euphoria which swept over his body. 'I have never felt so relaxed before in my life. I felt aware of every nerve in my body. I felt sad too, because for so much of my life, I've been afraid to really let go.'

Norman Dean Radican says that while he knows of and admires the work being done by Chester Mainard, Joseph Kramer and other sex educators around the world, he says he does not believe mainstream men are ready for such work. In his view, most men he speaks to are still very blocked about sexuality.

The Rileys believe women can help lead men into sexual health. Certainly, with the rate of male mortality on a steep rise, helping men get in touch with their bodies can only be a very positive thing. And as a personal tip – the sex afterwards is absolutely worth the effort.

COMING OUT

'There is much to learn in life,' I tell my mother who simply doesn't want to know all there is to know. She says most things are better left unknown, or at least unspoken.

My mum is British by birth and her philosophy is very much part of the English way of life. Life behind the closet door. Stiff upper lip, and all that.

The qualities she admires include: decorum, discretion, good manners, delicacy, and above all modesty, none of which are part of my general demeanour and certainly not part of my column, she often reminds me.

She also reveres neatness and as I am visiting Melbourne for the weekend, she has dragged me off to her hairdresser to have my scruffy, untamed hair cut into shape.

The salon – situated in the middle-class *borscht belt* of Melbourne – is run by two crazy gay guys, though no-one really admits they are gay. The clientele, mostly discreet, elegant ladies in their senior years, ignore the posters of muscled young boys that line the spaces between the mirrors.

They ignore the little comments like: 'Ooooh what a spunk,' when a young man wanders past the window, and make no mention of the fact that Trevor often wears earrings and make-up to work.

Not me. As Mother sadly knows, I never ignore anything. And last time she dragged me there, I couldn't help prising information out of Rodney and Trevor about their infinitely fascinating sex-lives. How often? How much? or simply: How?

'Stop asking such outrageous questions,' she huffed at me as I tried to discover everything you ever wanted to know about being gay but had no-one to ask. 'You are a disgrace,' she muttered as I interrogated Rodney about his former marriage and his coming out.

'You have no discretion at all! You don't even know the meaning of the word privacy! Well how could you, airing all your business in the paper every weekend?'

My mother is very fond of Rodney and Trevor. She is not the slightest bit fazed by their homosexuality. She just doesn't want to know the sordid details. Which is all I ever want to know. Sordid details and more sordid details. The sordid bits are the intoxicating spice of life. They also bring one closer to the truth. If you want to know how someone really thinks and feels, you have to know about the raw, exposed bits. The bits that are not on public display. The bits in the proverbial closet. The bits my mother sees as private.

Anyway we walk into the salon. Immediately my mother pushes me in front of the old Italian and Jewish women sitting there. 'Here is my beautiful daughter,' she brags as they coo, smile, and launch into their own interrogations: 'Are you married?' 'Will you have babies?' My mum answers for me because nice questions are not prying. I smile sweetly, the perfect child. Every mother's dream. Pleasant as a picture.

Half an hour later I am having my hair blow-waved by Rodney. I can't hear how loud I am speaking: 'So do you like to give it or receive it?' I bellow. My mother turns the colour of beetroot. I can see her in the mirror and realise I am speaking too loud. All the women are straining to hear what they have never had the audacity or opportunity to ask.

'I love to give it. Wouldn't you?' bellows Rodney. 'My boyfriend is the girl in our relationship,' he informs me, pulling my hair with venomous delight. 'He ... she ... prefers it that way.'

By now everyone has popped their heads out of the dryers. It is clear all conversation has stopped dead.

'Brian, my partner, has been a girl since about eight when her father died. She started dressing up in her mother's clothes. Oh! She wore the most gorgeous dress last night. We had people for dinner. It was a long tomato-red dress with shimmering, red shoes. She was dazzling, divine, walking down the stairs. I was so turned on.'

My mother comes storming up. 'Enough, Ruth. Please. Have you no shame?'

All my life I've had to answer that question, particularly since I started my column. But the answer is as evident to me as it is to Rodney, who is now so proudly parading his identity to us all, having spent thirty years of his life trapped inside the big lie. There is no shame in being human. And there is nothing particularly private in the experience.

Doesn't everyone make love? Cry? Feel insecure? Have outrageous fantasies? Failures? Moments of loneliness and humiliation? Suffer confusion about their identity, sexuality or relationships? Why be ashamed to admit it?

We are bombarded by lies, of perfect people living enviable and perfect lives. Our role models rarely confess to their humanness because in our society, it is important to make others envy our lives to validate a mediocre existence that we were promised would be far more special. So we all end up in the closet, one way or another, unable to speak the truth. Particularly in Anglo Saxon cultures.

'I had my legs waxed yesterday, what do you think,' says Trevor coming over to me, lifting up his trousers and running his hand down his leg.

Suddenly Mrs Goldfarb says: 'Very nice, Trevor. You look very nice, darlingk. Make safe sex, Trevor. You don't want no AIDS, darlingk. You too, Rodney.'

And all of a sudden it's out. The truth. And ten relieved women have joined in the discussion. It is a cacophony of conversation. Stories about gay friends of their sons, questions galore as fears and misconceptions are aired. The room is bubbling with a rare sharing and honesty, rare even for a hairdressing salon.

Some fabulous stories are offered by the women in exchange: confessions about sex after seventy, secret lovers. Rodney and Trevor have gone wild at the attention, the acceptance. Even my mother is drawn in at last to the real, messy and very indiscreet world of humans. What a joy. What a liberation! We are all out of the closet at last!

LETTERS

Dear Ruth,

For those ladies out there whose men are having problems getting an erection, buy one of those small, studded leather dog collars from a market and strap it on at the base. Be quick, the response is unbelievable.

ANON., QLD

Dearest Ruth,

You mentioned men having 'ball tucks' or scrotum tightening operations, to make testicles look firmer and more inviting. Inviting testicles! Isn't that a contradiction in terms?

LORRAINE, MARCOOLA BEACH, QLD

Dear Ruth,

Why are condoms so annoyingly big? They remind me of being a child at about eight, playing dressups in my father's clothes. You couldn't take two steps without your strides falling down. Having a small penis does have its problems. Someone wrote to you suggesting using the tongue as a great alternative. For whom? It isn't exactly a culinary delight – peaches and cream it ain't.

R.S., SYDNEY, NSW

Dear Ruth,

I am an old-age pensioner who thinks this generation's morals are going to the dogs because of its promiscuity, but for the life of me I really can't see why some people consider oral sex as depraved and unhealthy. Surely merely talking about sex has more virtue than actually participating in it.

GORDON, CLONTARF, QLD

Dear Ruth,

I was cosily reading your segment on Sunday whilst my fiancé was snoozing heavily beside me. So I asked him: 'What do you like better than sex?' Straightaway he said: 'Driving my boat really fast over the waves' – without even changing his sleepy facial expression. You had to be there! Love your column.

ROBYN, NOOSA JUNCTION, QLD

Dear Ruth,

SNAGs never get anywhere in their relationship with women. Eventually, the day arrives when the woman will sit the man down, and in her best intimate, communicative mode possible, start the conversation with...'You're a nice guy, but...'

DON'T CALL ME A NICE GUY, NT

Dear Ruth,

I have a noticeably bent dick. Of course, it was the subject of much name calling and hysterical laughter at boarding school in the showers – all very cruel. But my parents assured me that 'everything would be all right on the night'. This proved true. When erect it curves upwards and contacts the female's G spot more readily than a straight penis. I certainly haven't had too many complaints from women, just a gasp of horror when I drop my trousers.

MR B., ARRAWARRA BEACH, NSW

CHAPTER THREE

HOT & SWEATY IN BETWEEN:
The new androgyny

WHILST in New York, putting together pieces for my chapter on the new female sexual revolution, I spent a lot of time visiting clubs for women. As I explained in my first chapter, many were clubs where women of all sexual persuasions could go for a dance and a good time.

But one night I stumbled into a club that wasn't so welcoming. A quick look around the room told me that this was a club for gay women. 'Bull-dykes' was how a lesbian friend of mine later described the women who frequented this particular watering hole. My friend was not surprised by what followed given that the women who run this club are notoriously rigid. Not only is it an exclusively gay club, but only a certain type of lesbian need apply – your classic 'butch' lesbian.

In the other clubs I had visited, it was impossible to tell straight women from bisexual women or gay women. There was a celebration going on that blurred the lines. But in here, the name of the game was politics. The women all sported a sort of uniform: shaved or cropped hair, tattoos, pierced things, torn-off T-shirts and faded denims – in what seemed to be a statement against having to look erotic or sensuous in any way.

I ordered a drink and was immediately approached by a gaggle of really tough-looking broads who took me for either a straight woman, or a 'lipstick lesbian' which I was to discover is even worse.

'We don't want your kind in here,' one of the rougher dykes growled at me as the others formed a circle around me.

'What is my kind?' I asked in genuine curiosity, as more angry women surrounded me in an ominous manner.

Having discovered that to New Yorkers there is nothing quite as fascinating as an Australian accent, I did my best-ever Australian-girl-lost routine. 'I'm just new around here. I just wandered in here by mistake,' said I, looking sweet as cherry pie.

'Oh, you're from Australia?' one woman in truck-driver chic roared with great enthusiasm. The girls all seemed to relax. I wasn't threatening their territory. I wasn't one of those contemptible sorts – part of the trendy new movement to make lesbianism a hip fashion statement. I gathered they got a lot of 'that kind' in the club – femme dykes with big hair and jewellery that wasn't stuck through their faces, who believed that they could be whatever they wanted, or drink wherever they pleased.

I was curious to know how they immediately picked me as 'the wrong kind'. I knew the long hair was a dead giveaway but I was wearing jeans and a white T-shirt. I hardly looked that much different.

'The lipstick,' said one. 'The handbag,' said another whilst they all gleefully poked at my handbag. 'The way you held your glass of beer!' they laughed, very amused by this stage as they parodied the way my little finger shot into the air in a most feminine, and delicate fashion.

'The way you sit on the stool,' said a woman who was straddling the stool like a horse. I looked down at my crossed legs with horror. And then with even more horror at my white high-heels. 'Minnie Mouse shoes,' mocked one woman in heavy, black, army boots. The rest of them, all in military boots, fell about roaring with mirth.

After a while an odd bonding started happening. I told them what I was writing about. They explained to me why they were so agitated by the new breed of lesbians, many of whom condoned sleeping with men. 'They want to come in both doors but they don't pay at either end,' one of the older dykes sniffed resentfully, telling me about the struggles and battles the old-guard had to fight in order to be accepted as lesbian.

'They use us for experimentation,' huffed another. The pain in the room was palpable. It was clear that these women believed lesbians had to be committed to one way of life only. There was one way of dressing. One way of acting. One way of existing. You used language to name yourself: 'I am a butch. I am a leather dyke.' And then you lived under the noose of the proclamation for the rest of your life.

The new breed of lesbians have broken the mould of language. Famous lesbians including Camille Paglia have started pushing off the shackles of role, allowing themselves to be lipstick lesbians one day and butch the next. I've already mentioned how Paglia has gone further than most others, writing recently about her fondness for the penis. Other lesbians have talked of maybe getting married one day and having kids, some confessing to having slept with men and having enjoyed the sex.

The feeling of confinement in this club reminded me very much of the straight world – where we call ourselves something and then live under that tyranny. Women particularly have always defined and confined themselves: 'I am a mother', translation 'I am therefore clean-living, responsible'. 'I am a career woman', the connotation being 'cold', 'unable to nurture'. Men have never suffered these word shackles to the same degree.

For indeed language imprisons us. The minute we pronounce ourselves as something, we are then forced to behave in a way that is in keeping with that illusion.

The feminist ideology and political correctness of recent years has only further narrowed our options of what it is to be a woman.

There are many things we cannot change. If one is born black then unless you are Michael Jackson you remain black. You will always be Italian. At least by birth. But sexuality is not something we need limit. It can be a fluid experience. We have every opportunity to experiment and evolve our sexual personas and identities over the course of our lives – from submissive to dominant, kinky to vanilla, straight to bent. Sexuality as a journey not a given. As gender is a journey, not a given.

This is what this chapter is about. The new androgyny. I have realised, that as the end of the decade draws to a close, we are witnessing, perhaps more than any other time in recent history, a fluidity of sexual and social roles. By this I mean that the chasm between 'male' and 'female' is fast closing. Men are becoming more like women in behaviour and in appearance, women are taking on all the characteristics of men from the boardroom to the bedroom. And advertisers, marketers, image makers and movie moguls – sensing the winds of change – are capitalising on the trend.

And so back to my dyke club. The women all wanted to know how I defined myself. In terms of gender. In terms of role. In terms of sexual identity. They were pushing me to explain what I was doing in their club. 'What are you really exploring in your book? Are you exploring us, or yourself?' asked one bull-dyke, narrowing her eyes suspiciously.

'Are you *a breeder* (heterosexual)? Are you homosexual? Are you bisexual?' the women prodded, all milling around, curious at this creature who had inadvertently wandered into their lair.

I had been asked this many times over the years, hanging out as I do with a very mixed crowd. Sexual orientation was once described as a continuum with 1. being straight, 3. being bisexual, and 5 being gay. Surprisingly, most of the seemingly 'straight' middle-class friends – male and female – I have asked over time have identified themselves as a 2, even a 2.5. I have never answered the question on principle. No free spirit could wilfully climb inside a prison cell of words and slam the door on possibility. Or maybe I have just never known the right answer.

'What are you? What are you? Define yourself...' the women affectionately teased and bullied. 'Heterosexual, homo-sexual, bisexual...?'

I sat for a moment pondering the impossible question. And then on that hot, steamy night in New York City, inside one of Manhattan's most notorious gay clubs, surrounded by a group of total strangers, I heard the answer come out of my mouth. An answer that surprised me and shook me to the core.

'I am sexual,' I suddenly said, realising that that was the most powerful and liberating thing I had ever allowed myself to say.

'I am sexual,' I said using language to suddenly throw open the door on my narrow life, on a narrow club, in a narrow world. 'I am plain old sexual,' I said, feeling freer than I ever had felt in my entire life.

GENDER BENDERS

In a series of controversial advertisements by Calvin Klein, a gaggle of teenagers parade their bodies in front of the camera. Dressed in a mish-mash of denims, overalls, and T-shirts, they strut about promoting a new fragrance by the designer. It is impossible to tell the girls from the boys.

The point of the ad is to blur the lines between male and female given that the fragrance is ambi-sexual. But although Klein has again proved himself the maestro of ambiguity, he is not the only one pitching products this way. A whole rash of advertisements, products, clothing and movies are flooding the market in a bid to appeal to the boy-girl or girl-boy in all of us.

I remember the shock of picking up *Vanity Fair* and discovering my favourite singer kd lang shaving the lovely Cindy Crawford on the cover. It was an infamous shot that got the world talking. I thought it was one of the raunchiest, bravest marketing exercises I had seen in a long time and sales of the magazine went through the roof.

Not long after I was sitting in a movie theatre watching what I thought was one of the most extraordinary moments in recent film history, Tom Cruise, with hair cascading down his back, scoops Brad Pitt up into his arms and with orgasmic zeal plunges his teeth deep into his *objet d'amour* who is quivering on the brink of agony and ecstasy thousands of feet above planet earth.

In another scene from the same movie, *Interview With A Vampire*, Cruise and a smoulderingly beautiful Antonio Banderas with long hair and longer eyelashes, gaze longingly into each other's eyes, inches away from an erotic kiss and a million miles away from what would have been acceptable Hollywood imagery a few years ago.

The homo-eroticism did not go unnoted by film critics the world over. But what has is the extent to which films, magazines and billboards are displaying and pushing a new cultural role model. The gender bender. The androgynous icon.

Whereas androgyny has always been accepted, if not mandatory, for rock stars and avant-garde fringe dwellers, it is now being picked up by the mainstream. Even actor Jaye Davidson who played the boy-girl in *The Crying Game* managed to score a lead in the recent mass market, macho thriller *Star Gate*.

It seems to me that as the behavioural differences between men and women are rapidly breaking down, the image makers are capitalising on our shifting consciousness. Or maybe they are further fuelling the flame. The connection is unclear, but the evidence of a complete repackaging of gender roles undeniable.

For the past couple of years Hollywood has literally been spewing out films in which women have taken on swashbuckling, action roles formerly reserved for males. Whereas Sigourney Weaver's feisty role in *Alien* was once regarded as extraordinary, it is now boringly commonplace to see gun-slingin', hard drinkin', hard livin' gals as is evidenced by the latest craze towards the female Western with Uma Thurman and Sharon Stone amongst the big names donning cowboy hats.

Recently, the trend to female androgyny in film has taken an even more extreme form. A spate of recent films out have the heroine doing what men do – quite literally. It's called lesbian chic, and it's androgyny taken to its ultimate conclusion. Just as *Even Cowgirls Get the Blues* is a film about women who are more than just friends, so too films like *When Night is Falling*, *Reality Bites*, *Sirens* and *Love and Other Catastrophes* throw up images of same-sex erotica.

Lesbian chic is spreading like wildfire in the fashion world with androgynous or sexually ambiguous images dominating the fashion pages of overseas women's fashion magazines.

British magazine *The Face* recently featured a cover with waif supermodel Kate Moss lying vulnerably in the arms of another supermodel Helena. British *Elle* recently put Nadja Auermann and Claudia Schiffer together on the cover beneath the playful headline 'Nadja and Claudia in bed'. The same edition featured a story 'Women Who Live as Men'. Naomi Campbell let it be known that she recently stripped for gay women at a New York nightclub.

Meanwhile the catwalks of high fashion remain a showcase for androgyny forcing one British commentator, author of *The Designer Scam*, Colin McDowell to comment that the current decadent state of haute couture is the result of the misogyny of top designers – most of whom are homosexual, or an expression of their fantasies about women as adolescent boys. In fact, in some fashion shows, tall women have been replaced by beautiful boys in drag as a testimony to this fact.

I have been very curious to understand the profound changes we are witnessing and the implications for us all. So I contacted a number of social observers to find out what is happening. Many told me they believe the increasing trend is as a direct result of power shifts for women, and hence new role opportunities for men. Some call it 'the new equality'.

But psychologist Desiree Saddik from the Canterbury Family Centre in Melbourne says the trend to androgyny reflects a new form of malcontent. As relationships between men and women fall deeper into murky waters, as the divorce rate soars, people particularly the young and impressionable, are looking for a new way of being, she says.

'It is a trend born out of suffering and unhappiness in relationships. People are saying "If I can't have the other sex then I'll be the other sex".' She says to protect themselves people want to be omnipotent. 'They wish to be everything – male and female.'

Feminist theorist and lecturer in critical theory and philosophy at Monash University, bestselling author Elizabeth Grosz agrees with Saddik that the trend is stemming directly from people's attitudes. 'The image makers are not manipulating our attitudes. The attitudes are guiding image makers,' she says. 'Androgyny appeals to something deep inside us.'

Like Saddik she cites dissatisfaction with conventional roles, relationships and ways of being as a reason for the trend. 'Androgyny is not new in history. We see forms of variation in times of upheaval and crisis. We are in crisis now, which is a good thing. The world as we know it is breaking down. Feminism is slowly achieving the impact and change it has agitated for.

'The trend to androgyny reflects more choice in roles. It is very hip, very cool, very groovy amongst my students and among youth culture to be bisexual. The image makers are playing on the demand for role choices rather than creating them.'

Grosz believes, 'The current spate of flirtation with the images of lesbianism is good marketing because it appeals to women's increasing image of themselves as the strong, active female, whilst still appealing to the male fantasy.'

She says, 'Androgyny is a clever strategy. Both audiences are attracted to Calvin Klein ads. Like Mapplethorpe's art they open up all sorts of opportunities and choices for us. But are we ready for the choices?' she asks. And can the sexes ever really merge? 'Men can't have babies and women can't impregnate,' so it's all very superficial, she warns.

Lecturer in sociology at Macquarie University, Gary Dowsett, says he believes the notion of androgyny is a very positive thing for both men and women. He is fascinated by the homo-erotic ads in magazines and on billboards that depict men as languid, sexual, sensuous creatures but which appeal to both sexes. Many straight men don't even know that they are being subconsciously aroused.

'In many ways what we are now seeing is a return to the '60s and '70s – the unisex movement that came after Woodstock, where everyone had afros or long hair, crushed velvet shoulder bags and wore caftans or flared jeans. But back then it was a political movement. Now it is a social movement,' he says.

'There is more fluidity of roles in society being explored. The rigid lines between homosexuality and heterosexuality are dissolving. The youth of today are asking who invented these lines? People are slowly breaking away from the notion of two sexes – heterosexual male and female.

'Meanwhile gender roles have changed. Women are no longer seen in ads doing the ironing while husbands mow the lawn. The definitions of what it is to be masculine are rapidly changing.'

He says that while it is difficult for people to deviate from the so-called 'norms' and what we've been conditioned to believe, the sheer volume of information and ideas filtering down from new technologies will guarantee at least an awareness of our options.

BACKLASH

In hot contrast to the trend to androgyny the blonde bombshell is making a comeback. Stilettos and kitten heels are back. Pamela Anderson from *Baywatch* is the hottest new role model for hundreds and thousands of teenagers in what social observers are hailing as a 'feminine backlash'.

Outraged at what some describe as the defeminisation of women the hyper-femmes are coming out to fight, says one fashion doyen referring to the sudden trail of Hollywood films like *Showgirls* which are putting big breasts and bigger hair back on the map.

Big bums are also making a comeback in this catfight. Everywhere you look over here and in the United States, there are bums wiggling, wobbling and bopping to the beat. The latest dance craze features wildly gyrating hips whilst many of the rock clips rocketing up the charts talk about the joys of large posteriors. Film clips feature well-endowed beauties flashing their finer points at the camera.

The fashion is big but tight, offered one social commentator I caught being interviewed on TV recently. Clothes, particularly on the west coast of America, are cut to show off the big bum. Shorts are shorter than they have been since the '70s, with torn-off jeans provocatively revealing plenty of cheek.

Meanwhile in Australia there is a continued interest in anything which celebrates the female form in all of its fecundity.

A brisk walk down shopping strips in any of the trendy suburbs of our main cities tells the tale of the image war that is
being fought between women who want to embrace the new
androgynous chic and the ultra femmes.

At lunchtime on a crowded Friday afternoon, I see two
young women sitting in a cafe on Sydney's hip Oxford Street
looking like they've just paid a visit to an S&M joint – leather,
chains, PVC corsets, cropped hair – all the latest accoutrements
of the 'warrior woman' fetishist look. Next to them a woman
is wearing a business suit over a transparent, mesh top. When
she moves to read the paper and lift her coffee, her right breast
comes into view. Her garments are part of the ultra-feminine
fashion range described as 'strip-tease fashion' which is
designed to show off flesh.

The trend to strip-tease fashion came into vogue when a
cutting-edge designer chose a New York strip-joint to show his
collection which included sequinned nipple caps, satin slips and
snakeskin clothes. Since then the whole lap-dancing, stripper
culture has won renewed popularity.

The reason why large-breasted, big-hipped, bigger-haired
classically feminine women in figure-hugging or transparent
clothes are asserting themselves so aggressively is not just as a
backlash against androgyny and the waif-like bodies which have
for so long dominated our catwalks and our consciousness. But
also against the startling news that top designers in America and
Europe have started using men in drag to model their creations
both on the catwalk and on the cover of leading fashion
magazines.

Rather than opting for the super-tall, super-thin female,
they have gone the step further and are putting makeup and
wigs on beautiful boys and sending them out in high-heeled

shoes to face wildly applauding crowds who are apparently lapping up the pantomime.

Indeed, in New York, on the west coast of America and in parts of Europe, it is more super-hip than ever before to be transsexual, lesbian, gay, bi, androgynous or 'gender mobile'. And that is what is being thrown up to the public.

Female rock singers are getting stronger and butchier en masse whilst it is rare to see a male on stage who hasn't got the marketing advantage of androgyny. 'Being straight' is out of vogue which has sparked what can only be described as a conservative attempt to put things back the way they were.

But it is not just a backlash against women that we are witnessing. Bob Cannell, professor of Sociology at Santa Cruz University in California and author of the book *Masculinities*, believes the trend to androgyny has also sparked a backlash against the new, more sensitive, sensual male. He believes that men's movies and boys' computer games are becoming more violent, children's films from Hollywood are pushing the same old stereotypes, and the large-muscled, small-brained man, is more popular the ever. It's Rambo, The Testosterone Kid, fighting back.

Social observer and corporate trainer Christine Maher of Celebrity Speakers does not believe that a return to the past is possible. 'The '80s were the time of the entrepreneur. The '90s are the time of the nice guy. And now we're moving towards the '20s, the year 2000, which will be the time of the twin.

'Those people who can balance both sides of themselves: the ying with the yang, the male with the female, work with recreation will be our new heroes in all aspects of life.'

One thing is certain, the gender war will hot up as we hurtle towards the end of the millennium. Women are going to keep pushing those tits and child-bearing hips onto centre stage, men will be flexing their muscles, as others fight to redefine what being 'feminine' and 'masculine' really means. Whether the tides of change can be stemmed by the backlash is yet to be seen, but it will be an exciting battle. May the best *man* win.

LETTERS

Dear Ruth,

To Anon., QLD, whose friend wears ladies' underwear. I don't think there is anything wrong with any fella wearing ladies' knickers. I am a married woman with seven children and I wear men's jocks, because I find them very comfortable. I reckon there would be many others doing the same.

MRS J. (FOR JOCKS), BRISBANE, QLD

Dear Ruth,

If a female decides to openly demonstrate the masculine side to her personality in public, by wearing male clothing, society accepts her right to do so. To many, she is making a fashion statement. However, should a male decide to openly demonstrate the feminine side to his personality in public, by wearing female clothing, all hell would break loose. Why do we have such double standards?

ANON., QLD

Dear Ruth,

I am a cross-dresser and without the support of my wife, life would be very hard for me having to hide an important part of myself. I want to tell your readers not to be afraid to confide in their partners. To be different is not bad, but to keep the real you locked away is not healthy. If she loves you unconditionally then she will understand.

S.H., BURWOOD, VIC

Dear Ruth,

I am a straight man in his early twenties who, although he does not wear ladies' knickers, possesses many items of female clothing that he frequently wears in public including PVC pants and a brilliant ladies' silver jacket that I have worn on innumerable occasions. I feel great freedom in being able to wear whatever I like regardless of whether society deems it appropriate for me as a man or not.

'B', ADELAIDE, SA

Dear Ruth,

To Anon., QLD, take heart. Your friend who wears ladies' underwear is not the only one. It is estimated that in Great Britain alone, there are 500,000 heterosexual married males who cross-dress either regularly or occasionally. It is a known fact that cross-dressing is a strong antidote for stress. If the wearing of ladies' underwear brings out himself then why not? He is not demonstrating weakness. Femininity is about love, loyalty, affection, gentleness caring and so on.

ALISON, SUNSHINE BEACH, QLD

Dear Ruth,

I want to tell your reader from Victoria this. Having been married to a bisexual man for twenty years, I would urge you not to go ahead with this marriage. Your boyfriend can't and shouldn't be asked to change his sexual orientation. Please save yourself a lifetime of heartbreak and unhappiness. I love my husband, but it's not a good choice to marry a gay man unless you want your marriage to be severely compromised.

MRS R., WA

CHAPTER FOUR

HOT DATES:
Confessions of a single girl

EACH week I get bag loads of mail from many lonely people wanting to meet someone. They give me their personal details in the hope that I will publish their letters. They pray that their soul-mate will just happen to be passing and will be attracted by this obscure beacon in the fog. Exposed and vulnerable they wait patiently to be discovered.

And every now and again I run such letters even though they are not relevant to a sex page – for a deeply personal reason. You see, I too was once a lonely heart crying out for my soul-mate, waiting for that one-in-a-million chance that *he* was passing when I was calling out from the darkened pages of newsprint.

It was a few years ago when I was writing a lifestyle column. I would often reveal my feelings and darkest secrets as I believe a writer must in order to inspire honesty in others, and expose the illusions of life.

But my hidden agenda was that someone would read my

words and recognise me to be his woman. Spotting my vulnerability and virtues, he would then come for me, or so the myth went. My friends all used to laugh at me. 'You'll never meet anyone this way,' they would chide. We'd all gone through the rigours of personal ads, letters, dating agencies and phone services. It never worked. In fact, we had all had a string of disastrous blind dates.

The column did attract quite a swathe of male admirers. I often received letters from men who sounded almost too good to be true. Having bought the hype for too many years, I dismissed the photos of good lookers, and the success stories, and waited. Then one day I received an unusual letter from a man. It stunned me with its honesty. It was a particularly brave letter. The writer was obviously in a lot of pain.

He spoke to me about his fears. He was going through a nasty divorce and was frightened that he had failed. He wondered aloud what being a 'successful' human being really meant. His nakedness jumped out at me and I even shed a tear as I am apt to do when my readers reveal themselves to me.

A week later the next letter came. He spoke of things I had said in previous columns. He had been listening to me very carefully. He offered his philosophies and talked as if he'd known me for ever. Though I was intrigued, I was also convinced that he must be a nutter. Despite the fantasy, I was suspicious of someone who could take such an interest in the ravings of a person they'd never met, particularly a journalist.

But I found myself waiting each week for the letters. And each week they came. I found myself carrying them around, laughing, crying, as this man's life unfolded to me. And one day, overcome with affection, I picked up the phone and did what

I had never done before. I rang this crazy reader and asked him out on a date.

'This is dangerous,' cautioned my mother. My friends all shook their heads in disbelief. I knew it was foolish and I was nervous. But I felt strangely compelled to meet him. I spent days wondering what he'd look like. Before he arrived at the restaurant we had chosen, I drank three straight whiskies. Then into the restaurant he came.

I could smell the waves of his aftershave before I saw him. He looked nothing like I had imagined. Though he was a beautiful man, he wore clothes from the '70s. The floral shirt was so loud it almost knocked me over. The flared trousers were a trip. It later occurred to me that he was trapped in some time warp as many divorced men are. They often dress the way they used to dress on dates, before they were married.

But it didn't matter. It didn't matter what he was wearing or what he was going to say next. Because my trembling body told me that I was looking at the face of the man I was going to marry. And marry him I did.

It gives me enormous satisfaction to tell this story because often I get letters from angry people who say they don't know how my poor husband copes with a wife who exposes her sexual secrets each week.

Well my husband is now my literary confidant. And he has gone from letter writer to letters editor, sitting with me each week and lovingly sorting all my mail.

He married me knowing exactly who I am. And this is the only definition of true love. Someone who loves you for what you are, not for what they want you to be. I only hope that by publishing a few lonely-hearts letters every so often, I can give someone else the opportunity to know love like this.

Together we have gone back to some of the stories I wrote during my single days and chosen the ones that most amuse us to put in this chapter. We particularly like my horror dates and the stories that elucidate the confusion and indeed loneliness of playing the dating game.

I've just finished reading a story about a girl who was so lonely and so desperate to meet the man of her dreams, she put herself in the window of a bridal shop so she could attract a mate. I know how she felt. I think there should be a street in all the major capital cities around the world where singles can stand in shop windows the way prostitutes do in the red-light district of Amsterdam, and advertise their wares.

How else are we to connect in this lonely world? It is a sign of the times that when I offered my readers the chance to have a few lonely-hearts letters published on my page, I was totally bombarded with sack-loads full of mail.

In the next two chapters I make the transition from single to married life. But as my final story in this chapter THE FLIP SIDE reveals, neither is a perfect world.

PSYCHOPATHS I HAVE LOVED

The dating game is fraught with unwelcome surprises. At first the male peacock, chest full of hot air, colourful plumage wafting in the sunlight, crows and displays his throbbing red Porsches to draw you into the dance of love. Then he woos you into the jacuzzi of life whilst taking you on a guided tour of his monumental intellect.

All the while you quiver in your high-heeled, come-love-me shoes, waiting, waiting, for the fatal flaw to be revealed. What's the problem? you wonder as you sip champagne and hear how much he loves to shower women with sweetness.

And then it comes like a shot of whisky on an empty stomach. The crack in the glass. The reality check.

Like a recent date – intelligent, funny, attractive, and very generous with his cash – who after two fun dates took me to his apartment to show me his etchings. The etchings were of himself. Big, massive self-portraits in every room. Photographs, drawings, paintings with halogen lights trained on the images in case it wasn't clear who you were looking at.

Then there was the one who loved theatre, opera and art. He was attractive and kind. He loved Italian cooking. He got quite enthused during our viewing of the video *Matador* which is a gory and intriguing bit of Spanish film-making. He admitted he liked the concept of death. In fact, he thought the necrophiliac in the film was 'grossly misunderstood'.

There was the one who used to iron his hair and the one who made a bizarre clicking noise with his mouth when he chewed food.

But my favourite reality check came with a man who I met at Club Med. There I was, lying on the beach quietly minding my own business. He came strolling by, with his plastic Club Med money beads draped round his hairy chest. Advertising his wealth like an old Indian chief. He had knotted them into colour sequence orange-yellow-red, orange-yellow-red.

I should have known. But like so many women of my generation, I was so busy waiting for the arrival of the prince on his white horse, for the eternal happiness I had been promised, that I could only see a golden halo as I looked up at his sun-obscured form.

'Hi,' he said, beaming down at me, all gold and beads and white teeth and sunshine like a big Inca god. 'Can I join you?'

I recognised him at once from some article in a women's

magazine back home on wealthy, available eligible bachelors.

He sat down next to me and bought me a drink, which meant that two orange beads were forced to run together on his necklace. He said he hated that. I thought he was joking.

He strutted about getting himself comfortable like a lyre-bird in full plume. He was very handsome when he didn't smile. He said: 'How many Club Meds have you been to?'

I said: 'This is my first.'

He said: 'I've been to Thailand, Acapulco . . .' and on he went listing every region of the world. I should have known.

But love was already getting in the way. Love or neediness, which are both the same anyway, for women of marrying age.

On the beach that day, he read me a poem he'd written that he happened to be carrying around with him. It was ghastly. But I was dazzled anyway. Dazzled because he was single and rich and intelligent. And he was good-looking if you discounted the nicotine-stained teeth. Dazzled because it was summer and I was hot and sweaty, and ready, so, so ready to fall in love. Dazzled because he wanted me.

By the end of the week we were lovers. He asked me to go steady with him when we got home. I agreed.

I should have known. But hope is a powerful smokescreen. The opiate of the female masses. I had noticed the colour-coded socks in the drawers. I had noticed the way he arranged all his clothes in the cupboard like a rainbow prism from white to black, and that he would wear only the darker colours as the week wore on until Sunday was black. I was amused. I thought he was funny.

But one day in the park he became angry: 'That's not how it is done,' he said scornfully.

'What?' I asked, truly miffed.

'That's not how you eat ice cream!' he growled. 'I'll show you the right way,' and he snatched the cone from my hand and proceeded to lick around the cream. 'Counter-clockwise,' he yelled, growing very distressed. 'Counter-clockwise! You must always eat an ice cream counter-clockwise.'

'Or else?' I asked, growing alarmed. He glared at me in shock, as if I had worn red on a blue day, or put his pink socks behind the brown ones in his drawer. I knew the answer. The same fate that would befall you if you stood on the lines on the pavement. The bears would get you.

Now you, my precious readers, may think I am an overly fussy woman. My mother certainly does. I am not. We all have dreadful character flaws. Skeletons in the closet. I know I have mine. But it's a matter of what perversions and idiosyncrasies can you tolerate. For instance indecisiveness has never bothered me as much as say selfishness.

Hence, I have always believed that the dating game should go as follows to avoid disappointment and wasted time:

'Okay, lay it on the line. I can see all the good bits. I can see your clear green eyes. I can see you know your T. S. Eliot. What's your perversion? What's the fundamental problem? How are you a psychopath?'

'Oh well, I am filthy rich but I can't part with a penny. I'm mean. I mean *mean*. I am so mean I'd strap myself to the wing of the plane to avoid buying a ticket. I'm so mean I keep bread for six months and just scrape off the green bits. I make tea without the bag just to save a few cents. I collect used bottles to get the one-cent refund.

'What's your kink?'

'Oh, I'm fine. It's just that I turn into a sociopath around *that* time of the month. For one week in every four I turn into

131

a swamp creature. A quarter of our lives together I will be a putrid, vile-tempered beast. A stinking, growling, horrid, mass of man-hating flesh. But I'm fine the rest of the time. What do you say? Is there a love match?'

I think most people would agree with me on this one. You gotta put your bad bits on display. It isn't that the perpetually-single expect our dates to have no flaws. It's just that we want to find out about them before we take our clothes off. That's all.

HOCUS POCUS

Women, I have noticed, will go to any extent to net the man they love, the *objet d'amour*. Which is why love potions and voodoo dolls are doing such a roaring trade at the moment through reputable retail outlets.

Forget sexy lingerie and heady perfume. There are packages women can buy that teach them how to cast spells and catch dreams. There is even a marriage voodoo doll on the market to leave under the pillow at night.

I read recently that there are over 40,000 people in this country who admit to practising a form of magic or witchcraft. I believe a huge percentage of them are women searching for love. I know this readers because – and I pray to Beelzebub my grandmother does not read this – for a time I was a witch.

I was a witch from the ages twenty-one to twenty-two running around in circles under the moon chanting Latin anti-hymns in an ominous voice.

The group I joined was a derivative of an ancient witchcraft coven that had become popular again in Europe at the turn of the century. Its members were committed to saving Mother Earth. The modern equivalent is the anti-logging, dolphin-talkers, many of whom are also white witches or Pantheists. There are large communities of them living in mountainous, spiritual, regions around the country.

Anyway I must confess, that like some of the people I met through the coven, my motives were not pure. I joined not to save the planet but for one simple reason. 'D'. He was my English professor at a Melbourne university where I was studying for a year following my cadetship with *The Age* newspaper. I loved him. He was oblivious of me. Classic stuff. But I had to have him.

In class he taught us about the poet Yeats who was a member of a white-magic Cabbalistic coven and who used the symbols in his poetry. In art history class I was studying Kandinsky who was also a member of the same cult of mystics. What was the Universe trying to tell me?

I found out when I started dating 'N' who one night, after Chinese dinner, revealed he was a warlock and that there was a white-witch coven on campus. It all made cosmic sense. I would draw 'D' to me by hocus pocus. I thought all my black sabbaths had come at once.

This is still a time of youth you understand, when people tend to believe they have some control over the order of things, can change the world, can make people love them. Youth, when people still believe they and their lives are special in some magical way.

I had grown up on a diet of *Star Trek*, *The Outer Limits*, the *Twilight Zone*, *Bewitched*. There was magic out there: new galaxies and exotic creatures, men who were wise and beautiful and honest like Captain James Kirk. There was another dimension full of strange beings. There was power over one's destiny for those who possessed magic objects. I was still clinging to these hopes even though the years I had spent as a cadet journalist focusing on world chaos, steeped in the routine of finding parking spots and working off fat thighs, all hinted that this may not be the case.

But I wanted it to be the case, desperately, like so many who were drawn into the sect. For I have never since met such a group of misfits. Our 'temple' – for want of a better word – was inhabited by the fattest, saddest souls I had ever encountered. People who could not string a sentence together, who looked like walking zombies, who had been abandoned by parents, unemployed, helpless, hopeless. All looking for the magic, all looking for love.

Night after night I would listen to their unmagical stories of abuse and loneliness while we would wobble around in ritualistic circles, make the sign of the pentacles in the air, and believe in the forces of Nature. 'K' was 'in a bad relationship scene' with a woman who did not appreciate his midnight mass sessions. 'E' was an alcoholic. Some 'witches' were students, others just drop-ins from Beelzebub knows where – off the street I guess.

It took two years of devotion to gain admission into the inner sanctums of the sect. But just about anyone could participate in early ritual. The 'temple' itself was a clapped out, draughty, old warehouse in the outer suburbs with mystical signs painted childishly on the peeling walls. I was always too cold to go naked under the thin black robe, so I always kept my black skivvy and stockings on underneath, frightened that our leader would – through his third eye – see my deception. He never did.

The candles always went out from the draught so we settled for desk-lights with red rags thrown over them for effect.

Because most of us were unemployed or poor, we made do with a cardboard, fold-a-way, pentacle and a plastic chalice. Our leader was an obese hippie in his thirties. His wife could 'channel' and become other people. Sometimes, he told me looking worried, she would become someone else and disappear for days on end – with other men. Off in a puff of smoke! Magic is a bit like that. Precarious stuff really.

My mother caught me once on the veranda singing long words beginning with 'Omni...' and making the sign of the pentacles with my hand. She thought I was singing a rock song and doing some new dance craze. She left me alone.

I studied Tarot cards and dream symbols, and for a short, blissful, while, had a majestical purpose to my life.

Sex came into it. The group believed that through sex-magic and controlled orgasm you could project love and positive energy into the world, a sexual philosophy not dissimilar to those of Eastern religions. I really think that that's what a lot of them were there for. But I never practised sex-magic with the cult members. I was still very much of the physical world, unable to go beyond the blubber and large, hairy beards, and hopeless eyes of these bewildered people.

And I had 'D' – the incarnation of beauty, wisdom and eroticism – who one day toppled off his lectern with fatigue and didn't come back for the rest of the year.

I grew disgruntled, sad, unable to eat. It was not the ultimate loss of 'D', rather the loss of that magic object from childhood that I mourned. I guess, in retrospect, that is as good a definition as any of growing up. Realising that you can't always have what you want, that there is only this dimension, and the only reality is what you see before you.

I recently stood on a remote beach where a spacecraft was

believed to have landed, looking up at the night sky and hoping to catch a glimpse of one. Hoping against logic to be one
of those unique souls snatched away from domestica by little
green men and taken to exotic new galaxies. 'Beam me up,
Scotty before last night's dishes have to be washed and the bills
paid.'

I know I will spend the rest of my life staring up at the sky
waiting for Captain Kirk. But as I grow older I am learning that
the real magic is not in the outer limits. It is in being able to
accept and enjoy this frightening, uncertain and often precarious existence, the way it is. To treasure what you've got. And
ultimately, to stop yearning for what or who you cannot have.

DINOSAURS

As the world changes and progresses so quickly, it is nice to
know there are still bastions of civilisation that have not altered
at all. Where backward thinking is a way of life. Places which
haven't been ruined by New Age hog-wash such as a vicious
rumour someone spread that women were equal to men, and
were useful as more than sex objects.

The charming old world I speak of is the nightclub scene
of Australia which still adheres to traditional values.

Yes, here, under the strobe lights – hunting ground of the
old-fashioned sleazebag and the native greaseball – it is refresh-
ing to rediscover yourself for what you really are. No highbrow
intellectual. Just a walking pair of tits.

Out of interest myself and a childhood girlfriend returned
to the haunts of our youth, in both Sydney and Melbourne, to
see what had changed.

Along the way we discovered a host of new nightspots that
have sprung up in the wake of multiculturalism – Greek clubs,

Spanish joints, even an all-black African disco in Melbourne, jam-packed with people in dreadlocks. The new haunts were as delightfully 'traditional' as the great Aussie discotheque.

For instance, at a Spanish club I visited, I met a charming, old-fashioned type called Carlos who reminded me of my purpose in the scheme of things.

I had gone to see the Flamenco dancing the place is famed for. As I watched the show, I could see Mr Cool watching me. He stood against the wall. His hair was dyed black and severely blow-waved (or it could have been a hairpiece. I didn't want to look too closely).

He sported an orange shirt, open to the waist, a large gold chain and tight, tight, tight, black, flared polyester pants, a walking caricature of 1970s chic. He was chain smoking which probably accounted for the state of his skin: crinkle-cut.

I could see from his leer that unfortunately I was his type. I tried to ignore him. To no avail. I smelt his cheap aftershave before I saw him. Then he swept me up into riveting dialogue. He said: 'Hey beby, you wanna dance wid me?'

I said: 'No thanks.'

He said: 'C'mmon, honey. You dance wid me.'

I said: 'No thanks.'

He said: 'You very beaudiful. You Spanish?' I said: 'No.'

He said: 'You Aussie girl, Westie?' I said: 'No.'

He said: 'That's good.'

He grinned at me, revealing the nicotine-stained teeth he had left in his head, and after a few more slimy come-ons, he said: 'In Spain a man takes what he want. I take you.' Then he grabbed my wrist and started dragging me towards the dance floor.

Thankfully, a woman appeared who seemed to belong to

Carlos. On seeing her he immediately let go of my wrist and rather dramatically Flamencoed her backward onto the dance floor. She, drunk, stumbled backwards, tripping over her seven inch heels as he rammed her like a bull on heat. The testosterone seemed to flare in his body as he cornered his conquest. 'Olé!'

Carlos, was, admittedly one of the more aggressive types of traditionalist. Often these hunters are far smoother and more subtle in their approach to us sex objects.

Like the one that tried to pick me up at the African joint in Melbourne. I was getting into the Reggae with a girlfriend, burning off calories to the funky beat, when again, I noticed I was being watched.

Suddenly I saw some large man moon-walking towards me. You know, doing those little Michael Jackson dance steps. 'Oh no,' my friend and I moaned to each other as the prize cock got closer.

He was an older man. Black, with an American accent. He was rather elegantly dressed in dinner attire with a hat. The only problem was he glowed in the dark. He was fluorescent.

He must have sprayed clock-dial paint all over the white bits before going wooing. I guess it attracted the opposite sex to him in a way that being flat finish or matt finish didn't do.

He said: 'Hi, girls.' All eyes were upon this cool, presumably radioactive, daddy-o dude, who was obviously admired by the male throng.

I stared into his luminous eyeballs and then into his glowing mouth, crammed with huge white-green teeth. Then he started showing off, moon-walking his glowing shoes around us in funky circles to the beat, moving his fluorescent gloved hands in the air (to show what he could do to my body presumably) and tipping his hat, while other males clapped him on and said 'Ooooooow'.

I desperately wanted to laugh but I couldn't be cruel to a man so confused about women, so insecure, he had to wear clock-dial paint so I smiled politely and tried to walk away. But daddy-o was right on my tail. 'Where you from, baby?' he yelled at my back. 'Hey, girl. Don't be rude, sugar. Where you from?'

My girlfriend and I ducked into the ladies' and waited for ten minutes. By the time we emerged daddy-o had cornered another mama, a well-endowed blonde.

At a leading disco in Sydney I was accosted by many a dribbling beer-gutted male while at a Melbourne Greek club I attracted the attention of the head honcho who was smashing dishes everywhere. As each pile crashed to the floor he grinned at me, growing more excited and edging closer. His hairy chest oozed from his open shirt. Soon it became obvious he was smashing the plates for me.

'Throw,' he suddenly yelled to me, as all eyes fell upon me. Not quite knowing what to do, I picked up a plate next to me and as it hit the floor, the crowd yelled, 'Yasoo!'

'Yasoo baby, yasoo,' he yelled, taking my hand and dancing around wreckage. After ten minutes, no longer able to contain his profound admiration for me, he said: 'You wanna F...wid me?'

I like the fact that these old dinosaurs still roam the earth. It is good to go visit them occasionally in their native hunting grounds, because they are a good reminder of how things used to be on the outside, and how far we've come. Oh, ladies! Lest We Forget!

TOY-BOYS

At my thirtieth birthday party I was given a most unexpected surprise. Having suffered a broken heart, yet again, my friends thought I needed perking up. Specially since my mum reminded me over the phone about a statistic she had recently read: that a woman past the age of thirty had as much chance of getting hitched as being hit by a meteorite.

I felt down on my luck, until some close girlfriends announced to my guests that they would have to whisk me away at the stroke of midnight to give me a present that would lift my spirits.

The night was suspenseful. Everyone kept making jokes about what was waiting for me. Why did I have to be removed? How high would my spirits be lifted? Wasn't it something that could have been given to me in the restaurant? Could I eat it?

No, it couldn't be given to me at the restaurant they said. Yes, I could eat it if I really wanted. I was intrigued.

At midnight I was driven to a well-known luxury hotel in the city and given a room number. Because my girlfriends are delightfully sane and intelligent people, I didn't hesitate to follow their orders. They didn't accompany me.

After a nerve-racking ride up in the elevator I knocked on the door. A very handsome man answered and led me inside. He had a large bow on his lapel with a birthday card attached. The card had a use-by date: WITHIN 24 HOURS. Inside the card my friends had written: REALITY CAN BE BETTER THAN FANTASY.

I stood there in total shock, my mouth quivering with amusement, anger, surprise and embarrassment. This Robert Redford clone with cleft chin and blond hair had a bottle of French champagne sitting in a bucket of ice. He smiled at me and began to chat about the weather, the hotel, while I knocked back a few drinks to steady myself.

I really wanted to collect my bag and coat and dart out of there. But the weirdest feeling of obligation kept washing over me. I figured my friends had all put in a considerable amount of money to get the room, the French plonk and the toy-boy to cheer me up on my birthday.

I knew I had to stick around for a short while, if only to justify some of the expenditure. Also I was very curious to find out how the whole thing had come about.

After regaining my composure I ascertained that Mr Redford was actually a professional man who did some 'call-boying' at nights. Just to earn a bit of cash. His business had gone under in the late '80s and he drove a taxi, and offered himself to horny, often corporate women as an escort to help ends meet, so to speak. He was an excellent masseur he assured me having trained in several Eastern disciplines.

I felt myself growing more curious, particularly since I like cleft chins. They sort of make me want to put my tongue in, and twirl it around.

But I was still far too embarrassed to twirl, and being an intuitive kinda guy he reassured me that it was fine to just talk and drink champagne if that's what I wanted. Occasionally his female clients just needed to 'unburden' themselves or talk it out. Some just wanted company when they went to corporate events. Others, of course, wanted more.

Oddly, I suddenly felt a surge of pride. It was wonderful to think that women were now moving into the erotic domain of men. That women having now clawed their way up the greasy pole, having now reclaimed some of the power, were exploiting its potential. I had never adhered to the generalisation that women always wanted 'nice', meaningful sex.

He agreed that plenty of women liked it wild and raunchy,

or uncomplicated and without the sweet icing on top. Plenty of women had moved beyond 'erotic' – the tag always given to female sexuality – into 'hard core'. The thing about escorts that was so enticing to women, he explained, was that the men always wore condoms and were far more conscious of safe sex than your average one-night stand.

'If the ladies are still a bit nervous, I can always just give them a massage,' he said, cocking his eyebrow at me.

'Mmmm,' I said, staring into his cleft chin and wondering...

When I told my other friends about my birthday present they were outraged. The mere fact that I had spent the evening with an escort, regardless of what I had or hadn't done, was considered shocking, unbelievable, or just plain bad.

But I was interested to read recently that the trade in male escorts is now thriving in Australia. New services catering for female clientele are opening all the time with men charging themselves out at anything from $50 to $150 an hour.

As women's sexual appetites grow, the stigma on having these appetites decreases. Sex-shops for females are burgeoning around the world. Women are out of the erotic closet and into a whole range of specifically tailored products: soft porn, dildos shaped like whales, snakes and goddesses, vibrators shaped like butterflies.

Basically women are evolving their own sexual language and expression and the trend to escorts, and toy-boys, is part of this new sexual evolution. The best thing about it is that single women who are lonely and frustrated, no longer have to sit at their birthday parties crying into their beer.

Indeed not. Although I'm not the kind to pay and tell, from what I have gathered, the only crying they will be doing, will be crying for joy.

WHEN YOUR NUMBER'S UP

As a young, single girl, I was always looking for reasons to explain away my loneliness and the sad break-ups that I used to endure with frightening regularity.

I kept my head above water by rationalising that there was some cosmic significance to it all – that it was my destiny to suffer romantic deprivation in preparation for that special man who would chance along one day soon.

To help matters along I would often frequent soothsayers, psychics and the like who would counsel me in matters of Fate and how I could use it to find love. 'Go to Paris, he awaits you there,' offered one. 'He is close by. Perhaps he even lives next door,' contradicted another a week later.

One day, fresh from a bout of romantic disappointment, I went to consult a man reputed to be one of the most respected numerologists in the world. I needed to know where to be, and how to prepare for the big moment of 'falling in love'.

Rohinini was a psychic who could tell a person's destiny by adding up their birth date. He used a system based on ancient wisdom, tracing his knowledge of 'the spiritual properties of numbers' back to formulas from measurements of King Solomon's temple and the pyramids of Egypt. Friends had told me he was so accurate it was 'totally scary'.

Most fortunately, this maestro of the supernatural was based in our very own Australia. I sat in the lounge room of his little flat blowing my nose and lamenting the pain of love gone wrong. Rohinini soothed me with words of cosmic sympathy while he tallied up the figures.

'Oh wow. That's it! You are a nine. That explains it.'

My heart was thumping. I knew there was a reason my life had turned out the way it had.

He said: 'Nine...wow! God, that is such a special number.' And then went on to talk about me in a way that gave me chills up my spine. 'You are always searching for meaning. You feel frustrated because the meaning of life keeps eluding you...'

'Yes, yes...Oh yes.'

'There is a lot of sadness around love for you because reality never matches your expectations.'

'Yes, yes...how true.'

'But you will meet someone very soon. I can see him. He is tall and handsome. A man involved in money...perhaps a wealthy business tycoon. He will seek you out.'

'Oh, Rohinini, how can the numbers know so much about me?' I asked when the awesome session had finished. I was trembling. I wanted to kiss Rohinini's fat, thonged feet.

'They just know,' he said earnestly.

I asked him to show me how he worked out that I was a nine. He started adding up the numbers for me. 'First take your day of birth – 26th. Two plus six equals eight, then add the month, then the year. Remember the final number must be a digit between one and ten.'

'But that all adds up to thirty-five which is three plus five which is eight,' I said as he scrawled down figures.

'Oh...um...errr...eight. Yes. Sorry you are correct. You are actually an eight not a nine,' he stammered, turning red.

There was an awful moment of silence. Then he said: 'Look, it doesn't matter really. I mean, ummm, eight and nine are on the same grid so in reality they have almost identical traits.' He quickly tallied some new figures and said, 'That will be $45, Ruth,' and pushed me out the front door.

'But am I still special? And what about the handsome man?' I almost sobbed as he pushed me quickly into the street and into the grips of a cosmic identity crisis. There is nothing lonelier than losing your sacred number and your promising future.

I never received an answer from Rohinini nor did I meet Mr Handsome who was probably swanning around with some number nine.

I was reminded of this sorry tale whilst watching late-night tele recently. Amidst all the advertisements for telephone dating, there was one for some psychic hotline. Playing to the lonely-hearts audience the ad promised that people could ring up and find out whether love was around the corner. I felt a twinge of anger.

The next day I rang a woman I know who works for a similar service and she confirmed that for her it is all about being a good psychologist. 'You tell people what they want to hear. You sell them their dreams. It doesn't hurt them to feel optimistic that love is soon going to come their way. Sometimes it even helps.'

Someone said those same words to me recently when I told them how much I had paid for my face cream.

'Dreams in a bottle,' he laughed. 'You pay because you need to be lied to. You need to believe you're not going to wrinkle up and die.'

And was he wrong? If Rohinini had got his numbers right I'd have danced out on cloud 'nine'. In retrospect, paying $45 for a pair of rose-coloured glasses and a large dose of joy, was a real bargain.

WHO PAYS?

A few years ago, when I lived in New York, I was asked out on a date by a very amiable and pleasant-looking businessman.

We went out for a walk around a park and fed swans by the

lake. It was a charming afternoon, if you discount the fact I was bitten by a swan, and so I accepted a dinner invitation.

Through the meal we discussed why he was so screwed up, and why he thought he was not able to be in a relationship for very long, and of course, what his therapist thought. It was a meal that reminded me of an old joke: Now let's talk about you. What do *you* think about me?

Then the bill came. He picked it up and glared at it for a long, long time. A long time. Longer than I had seen anyone look at a bill before. I began to think that the meaning of life was written on the paper in invisible ink.

My date moved his docket-clutching hand close to his face and then further back, never lifting his eyeballs from the page. Back, forward, back, forward. Finally he pulled out $70 and put it in the tray.

I thought nothing of the incident. A few days later he popped in to see me on the way to an appointment and forgot his diary. When I went to put the diary in a safe place it fell open to the night of our dinner date because there was a book-mark inserted in that week.

There was an entry which I will never forget. It said: 'Had dinner with Ruth. Paid $70 for nothing.'

The proverbial 'penny' then dropped. The performance with the bill was like putting coins in a slot machine and then pulling down to see if you hit the jackpot.

My friend wasn't sure if he wanted to invest in an uncertain outcome and so was holding off paying for my dinner hoping that I may make some utterance that signalled an increase in odds – a more certain shower of gold coins like: 'Let's go to your apartment for coffee.' When I made him drop me off at the door, he felt cheated.

A week later, still reeling with anger, I accepted a dinner invitation from a sophisticated man who had the marvellous mixture of being both a lawyer and a novelist.

At the end of the meal he did not hesitate to throw his credit card into the tray, bragging about how successful he was. I invited him in for coffee. While the coffee brewed, he excused himself and went upstairs to the bathroom. He never came down, so I went upstairs only to discover him sitting half-naked on my bed – waiting.

Then came a sequence that looked like something out of a slapstick movie. He chased me around my room and down stairs while I yelled and threw things at him. Eventually he went home. He rang the next day to tell me he was never going to invite me to dinner again. He had never been so insulted in his life. 'You made me feel I was being totally rejected,' he yelled.

'You were being totally rejected,' I yelled back.

'Then why did you let me buy you dinner?' he huffed.

'I didn't think that taking a girl for dinner gave you automatic entry into her private quarters,' I huffed back.

I remembered a girlfriend of mine telling me that during a date with this man, he pushed her into a telephone box and kissed her brutally. This was after he bought her coffee and cake.

Things became much clearer for me once I had worked out the equation: one coffee equals one kiss.

I found that this formula was pretty standard when dating in Manhattan and eventually wouldn't let a man buy me a sandwich given that a sandwich could potentially rate anywhere between a coffee and a four-course meal.

In fact, nearly half of the men interviewed in a recent American survey felt entitled to pressure a woman from lightly to heavily for sex after they had paid for four consecutive dates, while a significant 43 per cent of men would stop seeing a woman if she had not 'delivered' by the fifth date regardless of who was footing the bill.

I found that because most New York women were financially independent, allowing oneself to be 'paid for' was often construed as just that, at least after more than one date. On arriving home, I was horrified to see that the problem was just as bad here. That awful question kept coming up. Who pays and what does paying mean? Because in the '90s men and women are as confused as they have ever been about where to draw the line.

Paying for dinner denotes something that 'going Dutch' does not. Implicit in it is a large degree of sexual politics, power and role-playing. It is impossible to know what your dinner guest's expectations are and trying to work it out subtly when the bill arrives is enough to give anyone severe indigestion.

Will a woman be offended if her date continues to pay or think he's mean if he doesn't? If she accepts does that mean there is romantic potential? Or that she is going to be a financial burden forever more? If she offers to pay half or insists on buying dinner, does it mean she wants to 'just be friends'? If he pays, does he have a right to expect anything and how does money influence the power-base of a relationship?

I have found that this confusion goes well beyond paying for dinner. Many of us, as baby-boomers, have inherited two strong ways of thinking: traditional '50s, and hip post-'70s consciousness. On some issues liberated people can regress back to childhood conditioning: 'This is what my dad did so it must be right.'

It is impossible to know which mentality will dominate any

given situation. The result is we often misconstrue our friends' motives, and feel hurt or rejected when our own expectations are not fulfilled.

The '90s are a difficult time for us socially. Men and women are not sure any more of what is *right* behaviour. Unlike our parents' times, there are no more guidelines or stringent moral rules.

'Who pays?' just highlights the mess we are in as we struggle to redefine our roles, what is politically-correct gastronomical behaviour and to work out what is really meant by the simple words: 'Can I buy you a coffee?'

MOVING IN

After a decade of singledom, moving in with a bloke – as in living together – can cause certain hiccups to one's lifestyle.

As I am clearly not the first to experience these minor tremors I thought I might ask advice from those brave souls who have trodden this path before me.

The most obvious first problem is how does one continue to remain glamorous and attractive to one's partner, indeed to retain the romance, in the face of such crushing intimacy.

Should one, for instance, be advised to set one's alarm for ten minutes before a partner's awakening so one can paint eyes onto the amorphous glob that has become one's face overnight?

Should one attempt to wash out the creases that have set into one's cheeks? Or does one allow one's beloved to realise that one's head tends to fold in on itself during the night?

If one's beloved's head has also caved in, particularly after a long, alcoholic evening, does one offer useful suggestions on grooming or does one pretend not to notice? Are dark glasses appropriate breakfast apparel? Is it rude to hide out behind the newspaper?

What about personal hygiene and sexual attraction? I once knew a man who kept a glass of mouthwash and an empty bowl by his bed so he could 'wash out the bottom of the dirty bird cage,' before his beloved reached across for a morning kiss. Is this extreme behaviour or is it to be advised?

Does one continue to wear the favourite, old flannelette nightie – a guaranteed form of contraception – with fluffy rabbit slippers, or does one buy a negligee and silk wrap? Are earrings a stupid or intelligent part of the breakfast apparel?

Should a man attempt to dislodge hair which has formed a plastered-down bouffant around the forehead and ears overnight? What if like a friend, he has no hair? Does he quickly put on his rug before she awakens or should he be *au naturel*?

A girlfriend told me about the time she discovered her man wore a rug.

She had come down to breakfast and noticed his face looked slightly bloated on the left side. She thought he may have developed mumps. On closer inspection, she saw he was wearing a hairpiece and had stuck it on slightly crooked. Seems he had been in too great a rush to secure the thing before she woke up.

One guy I knew used to sew shoulder-pads into his pyjamas to hide the fact he had no muscles. At what stage does one tell the truth about such things? And at what stage does one stop hiding the other things: one's haemorrhoid cream or potions for ulcers, tinea and sclerosis of the scalp? One's reaction to onions?

At what point does one cease from the exhausting process

of slipping into something more revealing or less revealing, diving into showers, into mouthwashes, into bathrooms, spraying scented goo on your body, around the room, trying to retain some semblance of dignity?

What is natural? What is gross? What is artificial, what is domestic etiquette? Because from this vantage point I have no clues. I have come to realise that whatever numerous and wonderful benefits come with the state called 'intimacy', there is little dignity in it.

A friend of mine who recently moved in with her beloved told me on the weekend that she lamented the loss of true privacy. She said that for many years she had snuck around her own home with comfort and security, looking ugly when she felt like it, sporting hair-curlers and sloppy joes. Enjoying her little depressions. Some days never getting dressed at all.

She always enjoyed juxtaposing these 'off' and slothful days with the excitement of dating her boyfriend. Buying a lovely garment, preening herself, looking and feeling beautiful after a few days of hibernation and relaxation from a world that poet T.S. Eliot described as forcing us to 'prepare a face to meet the faces that we meet'.

Now in this strange hybrid state called 'living together' she felt called upon to abandon both the romance of dating and yet also the security of marriage. She said: 'People are left revealing their most personal habits, leaving themselves open to raw scrutiny, without guaranteed acceptance. Ironically, what is probably needed to help commit-a-phobes make the leap into a heavier scene [marriage] is heaps of blinding romantic bliss.'

A male friend who has been cohabitating with his girlfriend for three years and is still unable to make the final commitment laughed and admitted that: 'Living together is like letting a buyer over-examine your second-hand car. If you let him take it for six days instead of an hour he's bound to turn up trouble.'

Using the same metaphor another male friend said he'd never live with anyone because: 'It's like if you bought a car and found it had faults you would rationalise your decision and convince yourself the problems were only small. If you hadn't yet bought you would be very, very, nervous about making the investment.'

Could it be our grandparents were right in hanging out for the wedding night?

I do ponder the wisdom of this strange thing my generation does, called living together. I ponder on whether it is better to know about the tinea before or after final commitment. But more importantly I ponder the fate of my darling, treasured flannelette nightgown. The last daggy vestige of my former lifestyle.

To burn or not to burn. To do the dishes again or not to do the dishes again. To split the telephone bill or not to split the telephone bill. To eat onions or not to eat onions. That is the question.

SEXY KNICKERS

Never, never, never, wear sexy underwear when you go out on a hot date. Because you will only ever get lucky when you are wearing big, ugly, bloomers with holes in them, and you haven't shaved your legs for three months. Life is like this.

The minute you spend $500 on a negligee, or some spivvy little knickers, you can kiss romance goodbye.

This profound wisdom has been passed down from woman to woman, mother to daughter, girlfriend to girlfriend, over the ages. It is a chillingly clever insight into the workings of the

Cosmos, adapted from early Greek philosophy by the female of the species.

Taken on a purely superficial level, it can be sound, practical, advice. But if one chooses to go deeper, it holds the entire wisdom of existence and destiny: the Universe is a random place. The Universe is cruel and merciless. If you are egotistical, show 'hubris' (human arrogance), pretend – mere mortal – that you can control Destiny, harness Fate, create your own Reality, then you'll be scorned and mocked by an uncaring, contemptuous Cosmos.

Better put by Shakespeare: 'As flies to wanton boys are we to the gods. They kill us for their sport.' Or my mum: 'Expectation breeds disappointment.'

My friend Elizabeth, a well-known journalist, recently conducted a year-long survey to verify this philosophy and discovered that 90 per cent of woman were seduced the night they wore pathetic, daggy, bloomers or bumble-bee stretchy pants with stripes. And those who weren't seduced in their bloomers were happy anyway, because who'd want to be caught out in that state?

The point of all of this is that I, like Shakespeare and the ancient Greeks, discovered the hard way that you cannot prepare for, nor tame, Destiny. Free will is an illusion. To pretend otherwise, to expect, plan, and plot, is to court disaster.

And thus said, I must report to my fans on my tragic undoing at my own hand – like the metaphorical self-blinding of poor old Oedipus. I did not heed the signs. I turned my head and wantonly behaved with hubris.

A month ago I wrote about my unexpected and fated meeting of Harry. Since this time, I have been flooded with inquiries as to how things are progressing.

Well, soon after discovering Harry on the Path of Life, I grew very uppity. I became rather self-confident, throwing in ancient female wisdom for the modern philosophical movements, telling my friends: 'I willed it to happen, I saw him in my mind's eye and put in my order. You can achieve your desired outcome. You can make reality fit your visualisation.'

Elizabeth, much experienced in the unpredictable ways of the world, got very panicky. 'Don't buy any fancy underwear,' she warned ominously, saying it was the female equivalent to a man carrying condoms in his back pocket on a hot date. It almost guarantees nothing will happen.

I laughed: 'Oh, come on. You don't believe that stuff any more? Don't be a victim for God's sake!'

She reminded me of her recent tragedy. She met a fantastic man. All rich and hot and panty. Things were really going well. Nothing awful happened, except for the night he got drunk and vomited in her car.

'Life is never this easy,' she pondered, feeling very nervous indeed. 'Will he die in a car crash?' But when he proposed, she suddenly forgot her humility. She was overcome with *hubris*, bragging to her girlfriends about what she had managed to achieve, gloating and floating and bloating up like a bubble fish. Within weeks he was gone from her life.

I listened to this with a scowl, believing it to be the stuff of negative thinking.

Not stuff of the '90s. Not the right stuff about taking responsibility and creating your own outcome.

And with that, week two of my new romance, I went out in a rage of self-empowerment and spent hundreds of dollars on lingerie.

I bought silky bra things and silk padded slippers and little lacy things that cost many dollars. The smaller and sillier, the more extravagant the price. Anything furry was over $100 and if you wanted transparent, add another $100. But damn the expense. It's an investment, I decided.

I lay around imagining all the fabulous erotic things that I was going to do in my silk muu-muu. I could almost feel his strong hands around my waist. I choreographed all the moves in my head. I took control.

At that very moment it was decreed. Harry would mysteriously take a fork in the crossroad that pointed away from me and my new private collection of transparent things towards another single babe.

Of course I am sad about Harry, but thankfully there are no signs of cancer or the worse afflictions the indifferent Universe imposes on those with *hubris*. It was a gentle wake-up call from above. I have taken my unworn lingerie back and used the credit to purchase some Italian saucepans and a baking dish. I'm back to bloomers, no expectations, and savouring each good moment – with gratitude.

GETTING HIGH

How do you maintain a relationship with a '90s person? It isn't easy because '90s persons have so many choices, they never know if where they are, is better than where they've been – or where they could be.

So every now and again you have to let your '90s person out of the cage to go for a bit of a wander, to sniff the greener grass, to amble freely in exotic new places, in the hope that your '90s person will get severely mangled by an on-coming car and come limping gratefully back. I mean this metaphorically of course.

Your '90s person will thus realise that the grass is not greener at all, just a little different. And, that wandering alone out in the big, wild world has many ugly dangers.

As I now lie here, with my foot up in traction, the bleeding, swollen mass of flesh tightly bandaged, I know that being let out of my cage for the weekend was the best thing my current permanent other could have done for our relationship. Not only was I metaphorically mangled by life, but my foot got quite literally crushed in the most horrible of circumstances.

The story goes as follows. On Friday night, I started pacing up and down the house with a snarly, irritable face.

It was the face of the '90s. The face of greed. The face that had spent the morning buried in glossy magazines reading about romance, adventure, and other people's exciting lives. The face that after many months in a happy, contented, committed relationship, wondered if it was missing out on something.

By Saturday morning the face was even snarlier. The jaws started snapping. By Saturday night my exhausted and long-suffering man opened the cage door and I went charging out with the girls looking for some action.

I had heard through the grapevine that there was a party on for single people. I thought that this would be a good place to prowl around, have a few drinks and stretch out into that sumptuous space called freedom.

It had been a long time since I had gone to a singles party. A long time since I had been out without my new man who I'd been seeing for the past three months.

It was an 'F' party where everyone had to dress up as something beginning with an 'F'. As I couldn't be bothered being anything special I put on too much mascara and went as Fabulous.

I was the only Fabulous there. There were three Fairies: two of them were women in frilly, pink skirts, hair in buns with wands, one of them was a bloke in drag. There was a Furry, a bloke with a fur jacket and a pair of cat's ears. There was someone dressed up like Captain Cook. I spent quite a while trying to work out what he had to do with 'F' until someone told me he was Famous. There were people in S&M garb, leather, lace and leopard-skin suits which led me to believe they just stuck on anything that would attract the opposite sex to them and they'd make up something 'F'ish at the time like Fetish or Foxy.

For a while I just stood around listening to music and watching a man in very tight jeans and a headband chat up one of the female Fairies. He looked as if all his 'F's had come at once until another male 'F' arrived, at which point the Fairy went twinkling over to him, threw her arms around him and began kissing him passionately.

Mr Tight Crotch went skulking away, deciding to take on a less challenging 'F' – a very overweight 'F' in a caftan. I meanwhile decided to hit the punch.

About five punches down I got up and decided to have a little dance with myself. The music was loud and throbbing and it gave one the tingling feeling of passionate nights on hot beaches in exotic places. The floor suddenly filled with lots of twirling, single 'F's who were all moving to the sounds of love.

My girlfriends had met two quite attractive 'F's and had lost interest in me altogether. This is the first rule of being single which I had forgotten. If you meet someone, you may dump your girlfriend anywhere, at any time.

'We're on the road to nowhere, come join the ride…' bellowed Talking Heads. It was great being nowhere, connected to nothing. Mr Hot Crotch saw me dancing alone and decided to

join me on the road to nowhere. 'I'm an ordinary guy...
Burning down the house...' came next. Lots of great nihilistic
songs.

'We're gonna get high, high, high, high, high, high...' It felt
great to be free. Great to be part of this whole 'F'ed party of
people going nowhere. I threw off my shoes.

Another punch and I was twirling in a glow of light. Round
and round then suddenly a shot of excruciating pain. I gasped
in shock not knowing what had happened. I almost blacked
out. The fat 'F' in a caftan was mumbling something about
being very sorry. I looked down and noticed a large hole in my
foot where her high-heel had landed when she threw herself
gaily into the air. One thing I forgot about people going
nowhere. They never look where they're going.

'Aaaaaach!' suddenly erupted from my mouth as I limped to
the couch and put my crushed foot up. I had to spend the rest
of the night on the couch with a cold glass of ice on my foot
waiting for my friends to finish with their 'F's and take me
home.

Funny how sordid and unappealing it all seemed from
down there. Suddenly Talking Heads seemed dated and repeti-
tive. The smell of fading perfume, alcohol and cigarettes was
making me feel nauseous. Mr Tight Crotch and other 'F's kept
coming over and making inane conversation which annoyed
me profusely. My foot was in agony. The fat 'F' kept shooting
me competitive looks which made me wonder if she hadn't
known exactly where she was going when she crushed my
now-bleeding foot.

I spent the rest of my 'big night out' worrying about
whether you could get AIDS from high-heeled shoes, and
thinking about my new man and how cosy and satisfying it

really is to stay home watching videos on a Saturday night with someone you love.

PAST PERFECT

We should never attempt to revisit the Past. We should leave intact its romantic illusions so they continue to match the lofty descriptions we award them: 'the best ever', 'the most beautiful', 'unbelievably wonderful'.

We should keep Reality's sooty hands from rubbing up against our inflated delusions. But we can't. We are a greedy and interfering lot, us humans, always hankering to go back to a time that was better.

And so, over summer, I revisited one of my most beautiful memory havens to recapture some of the magic lacking in a current brutal reality. I returned to Bali, seductive place of my youth, home of mysticism, exotic people and my own internal *noble savage*.

As a teenager I had gone there in search of adventure. I didn't want the deep suntan, sarongs, cheap shoes or Bali affairs that most went for. I wanted to explore the mystical heart of the island and the mountains where supernatural occurrences were the norm. I was always, in those days, craving the magical and special experience that would lift me out of the mundane, always waiting for the spiritual 'other world' to reaffirm that life was extraordinary.

'Seek and you shall find.' There he was standing on the side-walk in Kuta two days after my arrival. He seemed to find me, this boy, whose late father had been one of the most powerful and notorious magic-men on the island. He had long raven hair, and an eerie presence. None of the Balinese I had met knew quite what he did. He was a mystery.

We became friends. He taught me what I wanted to know. At 5am each morning we would go to the beach to meditate and sing chants to the rising sun. He took me into the hills to meet the magic men. They had bottles filled with toads and eels, used to cast a spell which brought fire and ruin to the cursed recipient.

I went to cremations, tooth-filing ceremonies, and coal-walking ceremonies, saw trances and shadow puppets dancing their dance of good and evil on the walls of dimly lit jungle huts.

My friend said he could kill a person by pointing his hand at them. I believed him. He and his friends one night returned looking frightened. They had seen a demon with a transparent stomach on the side of the road.

Despite the fact they tended to drink heavily and eat the hallucinogenic mushrooms that grew wild on the island, it never dawned on me their encounters could be anything other than mystical or divinely inspired.

But love is always a costly exercise – one way or another. The Balinese authorities were not terribly romantic and for each week I stayed beyond my four-week visa, I had to pay a horrific fee. My money endured for several months but finally the funds-of-love ran out. I told my friend I was going home. At this juncture he wept and begged me to marry him. Trembling and confused I mounted the plane intending to give the matter serious thought.

I never did. Safe back home I became consumed with the realities of financial journalism. I wrote many a pained letter to Bali but never got a response. I figured he was too hurt to write back.

So more than ten years later, I returned to seek out the remnants of that mysterious experience and find out what became of my Balinese magic man.

I found Bali more soggy than I had remembered it. In fact the rain never abated for a moment. Gone was much of the wild, jungle vegetation and sense of the primitive. Concrete stood in its place. Animal life consisted of busy colonies of Aussie and European tourists swarming the countryside.

I finally located a spokesman for the Past, a mutual acquaintance, and watched my illusions turn to waste.

Apparently my friend had married soon after I left. 'To another Australian visa,' the acquaintance laughed.

Seems my friend had been desperate to move to Australia, and had spent years before I had arrived playing up to the Aussie tourist girls. Another one came along within days of my going.

He and his wife had moved to Adelaide, to some working class suburb. He cut off all his hair and took a job working in a rubber factory.

And as if that wasn't enough to insult my beautiful memory, his job was to random-check condoms for holes. Another poorly-paid Asian immigrant on the production line of life. The power of the Past drained from my face. The Past should never be tampered with.

I spent the next week in Bali shopping, buying cheap sarongs and talking to myself a lot about life, and illusion versus reality. 'Ruth,' I muttered, 'at least you can never be hoodwinked again now that you are older and wiser. You can't be duped into believing in goblins and romance and fantasies and magic any more.'

And then I realised that that was the ultimate tragedy and sadness of growing up. That one could never recapture the magical excitement of the innocent and romantically deluded.

THE FLIP SIDE

My old girlfriend Lisa calls on the weekend to wish me Happy New Year. She has just had her second baby. She preaches the joys of child-bearing and married life over the phone – an annoyingly superior tone to her voice.

I am in the middle of teaching myself aromatherapy and reflexology, simultaneously, when she calls. I am massaging rose oil into my left foot while trying to balance the oily 'How To' book on the top of my knees and cradle the phone in my right shoulder. I groan softly to make the massage sound fabulously exotic, indulgent and decadent – the sort of thing that only 'single' people can do because there is no-one around to annoy them or make demands, or that need chasing with oily feet.

She wonders aloud whether she should read books to baby Karen at two months old : 'to feed her mind'. I wonder whether I have just massaged my kidney or liver or left eye according to the foot-diagram balancing on my knee being myopic at the best of times. Meanwhile the geranium oil, meant to 'induce a feeling of euphoric relaxation when it hits the olfactory system', has just hit the carpet which my room-mate, who hates 'incense-type things', will not be pleased about.

'I am so happy,' Lisa coos, inviting me to envy her nurtured existence. Two beautiful little girls, a wonderful husband who is sensitive, loves kids, has a superb income, all living together in their merry Edwardian home which they are forever renovating.

'I am so happy,' I coo back, dropping little phrases like 'travelling overseas again soon', 'writing a film script', 'met a gorgeous guy...', 'multiple orgasms'.

My life certainly does sound exciting as I hang up the phone and return to rubbing the frigging oily mess into my fat feet because I have nowhere to go that night, the phone having not rung all day.

Lisa isn't really happy either, I remind myself. I know because one winter night last year, after a few too many drinks, on one of the rare chances she has had to get away for the evening, she cried and confessed that she hated me. She hated my life, my career. The years I spent living in Manhattan and working as a journalist in strife-torn Israel.

She envied my ability to take risks. Hers was a measured, predictable, existence she said. Her husband was a bore. Her child drained every ounce of creative energy from her. She had moved from home to marriage without so much as a stop in between. She had never taken major risks in her life.

'You are Ruby Tuesday,' she spluttered from her wineglass. A blast from the past. I grew up in the '60s. I used the song as my role model. I used to run around as a teenager in hot-pants and love beads singing: 'Goodbye Ruby Tuesday, who can hang a name on you? And when you change with every new day, still I'm gonna miss you.'

That free spirit was always going to be me. 'Yesterday don't matter because it's gone...' Then one day that free spirit was me, as I pushed myself further and further out of my cosseted environment into uncharted terrain.

But Mick didn't tell us that Ruby Tuesday, drifting around the world trying to 'catch her dreams before they run away', spent a lot of Saturday nights at home alone eating chocolate bickies to stimulate her deprived hypothalamus. Because being a free spirit meant long stretches without relationships or sex.

He didn't tell us that spending every dollar you earned running around the world in search of 'something' that always seemed to have moved on just before you got there, induced a sour state of being called poverty.

He didn't talk about date rape and diseases like AIDS and Hepatitis B. Or about what it feels like to share your soul with some new guy, or girlfriend, only to have all that 'knowing' you have slowly built, evaporate, when the time comes to part.

Ah Mick, you old bastard. You fooled us all. You didn't give us the flip side of the album. You didn't state the cost of insatiable curiosity, greed and an inability to commit. I said to Lisa that night from my drunken stupor: 'Freedom is a selfish, empty, illusion (hiccup!).'

She said: 'Maybe if we have another baby we will be happier. Marriage is so dull. We hardly ever have sex any more. I'm so jealous about New York.'

I said: 'In New York I lived with a divorced woman who saw an analyst three times a week and had 200 shampoo bottles lining the walls of her bathroom because she believed that if she found the right shampoo her life would work out. She would find meaning.

'What is it you want that I have, Lisa? I'll trade it for a bit of continuity, emotional warmth, and meaning. For your ability to make emotional commitments, teach children about the world and care for them, to live in a home that always has someone in it.'

Her eyes grew troubled as she contemplated the shampoo bottles, the overall chaos of my life and the strange souls who inhabited it. Finally she said: 'Don is a good man. Our relationship will come good. It always does. We like being together. He can be very funny, you know. I do love him...'

I guess I must have looked pretty troubled at that point too. Because the dimensions of her life suddenly dawned on me.

Mediocrity has never been a concept Ruby Tuesday has been happy with. 'She just can't be chained to a life where nothing's gained and nothing's lost, at such a cost.'

So off home we went that night in winter last year, both satisfied with our own lot. And we've lapsed back into strutting our lives at each other competitively down the phone line.

I know Lisa gets bored. I get lonely and insecure. I know she gets sick of people making endless demands of her. I get sick of massaging my own feet, and ego. Don's face drives her mad at times. I get loco at the endless stream of new faces through my life as I search, search, search, for that eternal something Mick Jagger promised me.

I know also, as I go back to massaging my feet and mopping the oil stains off the carpet before my room-mate gets home and screams at me, that I am no happier or sadder than Lisa. Contentment is not a reality, belonging to a specific way of life. It is a state of mind. And the grass is not greener elsewhere. It is just different on the other side. Just different. That's all.

HOT & SWEATY

LETTERS

Dear Ruth,

I found that for the past eight years my blow-up doll was giving me silent pleasure, but it would be nice to be able to talk to a live person. As I do not drink, or go to the pub/club, I do not meet people of the female gender. I am fifty-three years of age, six feet tall. Is there a real woman out there for me? If there is, please write.

A., SOUTH SYDNEY, NSW (DETAILS PROVIDED)

Dear Ruth,

To A, of South Sydney. Surely letting down your blow-up doll after eight years is just a bad case of the seven-year itch?

DON, CASTLEREAGH, NSW

Dear Ruth,

The reason I blame for my lack of success on the dating scene is because of men's one-liners. As soon as a man opens his mouth I usually feel compelled to vomit. It's either corny ('What's a nice girl like you...'), pathetic or crude ('Let's go out for a feed and then back to my place for a root'). These things have really been said to me. Men are better off saying nothing at all.

DESPERATE, BONDI, NSW

Dear Ruth,

My son recently asked me what I thought about sex before marriage. I told him, 'Go for it, son, there is precious little after marriage.'

FRED, MT TAMBORINE, QLD

Dear Ruth,

I'd like to mention that why men don't bother to talk to women of beauty is that such women think their shit doesn't stink. Myself and my mates find it much easier to talk to a plainer Jane because she is friendly, open and relaxed with us. With the way equality is today we'll stick with plain Jane until the beauty comes over and asks us out.

D.A., PERTH, WA

Dear Ruth,

So there is a 'chronic shortage of straight, available male talent'. If this is seriously the case, then where are the hordes of straight, available female talent that is supposed to exist? I have become increasingly convinced that they are either gay, married, already have kids, men-hating feminazis or pining for that twenty-stone gorilla that treats her like dirt.

WAITING

Ruth Ostrow,

I was well over thirty before I had my first sexual experience. I had given up all hope of ever meeting anybody, so I finally telephoned a prostitute to visit me in my home. Despite all I had heard, the woman turned out to be a warm, happy and caring person whom I have asked to return once a month. Why do the police, the press and the public give these women such a bad image? To many lonely men like me, they are the only female company we will have.

K.B., BRISBANE, QLD

CHAPTER FIVE

HOT MONOGAMY:
A contradiction in terms?

HAVING now been married for a few years I look at life this way. When you're single, you are unhappy because you are always hot and thirsty with no water in sight. It's a perpetual desert with trekkers stumbling on the occasional oasis which eventually dries up. You dream of marriage and a time where hot and cold, free-flowing love is always going to be on tap. You will drink yourself into oblivion. You will drown in the abundant overflow.

Then you get married and it's true. There is plenty of water around. Gushing, shooting springs, clear pools of glimmering moisture, available, just waiting to be lapped up. The problem is that no-one is thirsty. Well, you might get thirsty every now and again but after bills and babies' bottoms and the traumas of domestic life, who has the energy to drink?

And so this chapter came about. The pitfalls of permanence. Life behind the picket fence.

I was not at all surprised by the recent results of a survey by

Deakin University in Melbourne which proves that most people in marriages and long-term relationships have far less sex than media hype would have us believe.

Almost two-thirds of the couples who took part in the university survey – an intense year-long study of marriage or live-in situations in Australia – had sex from once a week to once a month. A significant percentage even answered 'never', with the most recent findings from a News Limited survey putting the figure of couples who never sleep together at 10 per cent or a startling one-in-ten.

Meanwhile another study reported in the American publication *Journal of Marriage and the Family* showed that not only weren't couples doing it that frequently, but they weren't doing it for that long either. Apparently the average couple has sex for only fifteen minutes at a pop!

According to Professor Marita McCabe, the woman who instigated the Deakin University survey: 'Although 90 per cent of couples said that sex was important or very important for them, we have found that the frequency of sex for married couples in longer relationships, particularly for those over forty-five years of age, was around once a month.

'Those younger than thirty and in early relationships were the "several times a weekers" but that dropped back significantly as the length of relationship, and age of couple, increased.'

She tells me that researchers also uncovered that people lie 'significantly', usually to themselves, about frequency of sex. This is particularly true of men, who want to see themselves as potent. When interviewed, the wives told a very different story.

The survey forced people to take into account their *dry* patches and make an aggregate assessment, thereby admitting to the true state of their sex-lives. With all the information available to us about the effects of children, aging and stress on libido and sexual prowess, it's sad to see that so many people still need to see themselves as veritable sex-machines.

A lot of this chapter has been inspired by the rather dramatic changes to my own sex-life that I have witnessed since marrying, inheriting two teenage step-children and having a baby. I remain preoccupied with the eternal question: Can eros and domesticity survive together in the same house?

If they can live together then they are certainly not easy bed-fellows, as I have discovered in trying to keep my own marriage hot and sweaty.

But I flatly refuse to let my vagina die a natural death, although I can see how vaginas could quite easily suffocate and penises drop off, behind the closed doors of suburbia – without anyone even noticing. I guess when you think about it, it seems that I am one of those sad cases who wants to continue to be a sex-machine, despite the chronic lack of sleep from a teething toddler, work pressures and the general thrust and grind of life.

'Is it an impossible dream to imagine one can stay *hot and horny* whilst *married with kids*?' I ask in this chapter, as I drag my amused and ever-enthusiastic husband along to all sorts of strange and often hilarious courses and clubs, workshops and weekend retreats, sex-shops and strip-joints in a bid to learn the ultimate secret: *The Secret of Sex After Marriage*.

I wish you all many hours of *Hot Monogamy*. Well, it may prove a contradiction in terms, but it sure beats the alternative.

BABY LOVE

My relationship with my husband has altered profoundly since our baby daughter began to grow up and talk and assume a personality of her own.

Our conversations revolve around her – the colour of her hair in the sun, what she ate, how she ate, why she cried, how she smiled when we gave her crayons and paper. It is an obsession, our obsession – a shared, crazy, obsessive love that seems to bond us together like thick pasty glue, and yet it is tearing us apart.

We don't notice each other any more. I am trying to hear him but I hear only her, crying, demanding attention, or gurgling her happy sounds, the half-human language that keeps me mesmerised. I am transfixed by the sentences, the meaning of her own treasured words. To me they are the most intoxicating sounds in the world. I can listen for hours to her sing-song voice without getting bored. I am in a trance. He can't compete. Nothing he says to me means as much.

And I can't compete. Nothing I do or wear, or create, holds his gaze like she does. It is only her he sees – her in an enraptured state splashing in the bath, her in the back garden, her with food being spat out all over the table and then rubbed into her hair. He is laughing, scolding, cooing, cajoling. He is looking at her the way he used to look at me, as if his eyes can't drink in enough, and I am competing with him to drink in even more of her and snap these memories into my mind like precious photographs of the best years of our lives.

He sees nothing but her, I see nothing but her. We are desperately, passionately in love with her, and there is nowhere to go with this consuming love.

The experts say that children sap libido. I know it to be true. There is no room, no space, no time between work and her, and her and work and finally sleep which we grab gratefully at the end of every exhausting, fulfilling, happy day.

'Let's go for dinner,' I finally suggest one night after an

emotionally draining day of new toys and dance steps and *Old Macdonald Had a Farm* played over and over and over again until we are both pulling our hair out. 'I need to get away,' I say thinking of how much time has elapsed since we had time for intimacy, since we just held each other and loved each other and made love to each other and whispered secret thoughts.

At the restaurant we stare at each other through foggy, vacant eyes. We talk a little about him and a little about me and then the menu comes and it reminds us both of her and how naughty she's become at dinner time and how she says 'no' to everything even if she desperately wants it – the beginnings of the terrible twos, and we are laughing and sharing our love of her and before we know it the bill has arrived and we've spoken of nothing else.

I sit at my computer wanting to write a story about how children affect people's sex-lives and why. And instead of quoting the experts I am confessing to a love affair that is so overwhelming that we are losing each other, my husband and I. We are both stuck in a place that is so heavy with loving and caring that we're forgetting how to be together. I wonder how many other couples out there have lost each other in the murky waters of parenthood?

The experts say that couples with children have two to three times less frequent sex than couples without. The experts also say that two children are more debilitating to libido than one, and three more than two. They talk of the physical and emotional exhaustion of raising kids. They talk also of the impact new roles have on sexuality.

This is true. I see myself as a mother now, I see him as a daddy, and it is hard to see each other differently. But I insist we try.

So finally we send her to mother-in-law's for the evening. She is gone and we start to talk about her. I put a stop to it. I put her toys out of sight and pour the wine, and it slowly begins to return, the eroticism, the conversation, the closeness, the sexuality. It comes slowly then fast and furious. Because I have missed this man, my husband, my lover who became a father, and he has missed me.

And we hold each other and vow to not lose each other again in the milky love of parenting. But I know that it is not easy to be like this and it is hard to let her go even for a moment. And I know that after a child is born, we like so many other parents, will have to remember to remember each other for the rest of our lives.

SEX-MACHINE

For those of us whose sex-lives are more erratic than erotic, the survey by Deakin University claiming that most couples in permanent arrangements had sex from between once a week to once a month, is welcome news.

It finally explodes a nasty myth that we have all had to live with since women's magazines, television and Hollywood movies have started bombarding our lives with the quest for the perfect orgasm, the better orgasm, orgasm of the G spot, multiple orgasm of the nasal passage.

Many of us have laboured miserably under the terrible misconception that every other couple, including the neighbours, the milkman and his wife, and anyone in a hundred-mile radius, is having unbridled erotic experiences in every room of the house while we alone are influenced by the chronic ups and downs of life.

Pulp fiction, churned out each week in the guise of

'serious journalism', has led us to believe that we alone are depleted by exhaustion, anxiety, work, children. We alone are worn down by the endless demands put upon us each day from old or dying parents, sick children, the unsympathetic boss – the general 'coitus interruptus' of life.

The sense of inadequacy, unreal expectation or jealousy has been enough to make many people run off from perfectly good, normal marriages, in quest of this eternal bonking that we never seem to be getting. It has sent us into impotency clinics, to shrinks, to younger lovers, to hell and back with the question burning in our brains: why can't we manage it three times a month let alone three times a night?

And the sad conclusion that many people reach, if divorce statistics in this country are anything to go by, is: 'My marriage is bad. After all it must be my partner's fault I'd rather watch B-grade movie stars battle Blobs, Things and furry monsters with button eyes, than dangle naked from the ceiling covered in whipped cream.'

But the chances are, there is nothing wrong with you or your marriage. The statistics reveal that after a long, hard day, the majority of people out there in the suburbs of Australia would rather turn on the TV than themselves.

But though the average Aussie couple may not have the stamina nor time to go at it all that frequently, when they do bonk, it seems to be a happy, satisfying experience.

My own research has borne this out. When I first got hold of the survey I ran around to all my married friends showing them the statistics. The survey was met with jubilation and excitement. 'So we're normal?' sighed one girlfriend in what seemed to sum up the general response.

Talking to my friends over the years, I discovered that our

sex-lives waxed and waned with the weather and the degree of problems and time constraints in our lives. Our husbands' libidos varied according to daily pressures and very often what was on television that night. And it was fine with us.

After our first babies were born, we concurred that it would be preferable to be boiled in oil while eating a tarantula spider than have sex. We all fantasised about bed, but it was the doona we yearned for, to have its thick fluffy stuffings wrapped around our naked bodies while we drifted off to meet the sandman. My husband had to compete with bed-linen for my affections.

But we were happy. We had all had normal, healthy, sexual appetites before babies. And sex returned in time, as it always does after the various traumas and problems of life pass over.

One friend, Helen Rons, married five years with a toddler, admitted that she and her husband hadn't had sex for months when I showed her the survey. But she wasn't at all upset by it.

'Oh, it's quite normal for us to have either feast or famine. We can go at it quite consistently then just lose interest. Once we've lost interest, time just goes by with one thing and another. I sit up watching TV till late or he watches the tennis.

'But then we may go away for a weekend and we fall in love again,' she grinned.

The spate of recent surveys confirm a belief I have always held. That if you give most people the choice between okay sex very regularly or special sex less frequently, that most people instinctively go for the latter. After all, we all know what chocolate tastes like when we've been dieting, or how wonderful that cigarette or beer tastes when one is trying to cut down. It is quite logical to allow a few days or weeks to elapse in order to rebuild one's sexual appetites and allow for some 'yearning', an essential ingredient in sex.

When you think about it, all the sex we had when we were single wasn't necessarily 'great' because those lovers were better than our current partners. Rather, we had to wait so long between courses that we pigged out in wanton, blissful, ecstatic gluttony when the food finally came, raving about how good it tasted. And we never took it for granted.

In fact, a whopping 70 per cent of those surveyed by Deakin University were perfectly content with their infrequent sex-lives. As long as sex – when they had it – was exciting and pleasurable, the majority showed a strong preference for quality sex over quantity.

So despite the 'big-is-better', 'more-is-best' mentality we have inherited from American culture, Australians are still down-to-earth enough to vote with their bodies for satisfaction over performance to make sex the special act it should be.

But if the research filtering in from all over the world suggests the norm is quality not quantity sex, then why are most people still riddled with self-recrimination and self-doubt?

Why do so many men feel totally dejected because they can't get it up every night and keep it up for long periods of time? Why do so many women walk around feeling 'I'm lousy, I've lost it', or 'Our marriage has lost it'? The mere knowledge of which has sent us en masse looking for what it is we've lost.

It's because media hype never allows us to feel happy with ourselves. Whole industries have sprung up to help us get back what we *think* we've lost – selling sex-aids, beauty creams, clothes and cosmetics, holidays, therapists for mid-life crises. And it's in the media's interests, feeding off the advertising dollar, to keep pummelling the myth.

But the truth is that whatever it is we fear we've lost, we never had it in the first place. It is another well-kept open secret that eros and domestic life do not mix. And maybe they were never meant to.

It is impossible to discuss nappies and garbage bags with someone and then fall passionately into bed the way you did when you were courting. That's why for many centuries in Europe, before the Industrial Revolution, it was quite appropriate to take a lover.

There was the person you had torrid, unrequited love with, and there was your spouse for security and child-rearing.

Now we expect both in the one partner. We demand the challenge of the new, the erotica of romantic love, coupled with the day-to-day grind of making ends meet and rearing kids. But let's be realistic. Discussing the endless stream of bills, and family biological problems is not a turn-on. And glaring at someone's dermatitis cream and haemorrhoid lotion on the bathroom shelf every day certainly takes the edge off passion. Bills, boredom and bum creams do not an erotic fantasy maketh.

It isn't that you can't have both. The statistics clearly show that you can. But it's difficult in the pressure-filled '90s to find the time or energy to slip out of our domestic roles and into something more comfortable. Hence the frequency of sexual activity declines as the effort needed to create romance increases.

Doctor Debbie Then, a psychologist from the West Coast of America, summed it up whilst recently in Australia. 'You just have to look at personal hygiene to see what is wrong with people's sexual relationships. When we are dating someone we take the time to get dressed, wash our hair, put on make-up and beautiful clothes.

'After several years of marriage, many women let themselves

go. They don't bother to dress up for their partners any more. Men and women will often come home from work with bad breath, and smelly armpits. They're tired. They don't talk to each other.'

But she believes familiarity does not have to breed contempt. She says the couples who take the time to create an erotic side to their marriage and who make the effort to flirt with each other, are the ones who have a satisfying sex-life – no matter how frequently or infrequently they end up doing the deed.

HOT MONOGAMY

The course literature said that doing the workshop would help us 'unlock the child within'. We would be able to find our 'playful inner core' and reinvigorate our marriage. We would learn how to reconnect with our 'erotic fire'.

It was the final one that got me. Something very sad happens to one's 'erotic inner fire' after marriage and children. The 'outer garbage can' of life filled with bills and last night's chops, and nappies, somehow lands on top of it.

Although my husband loved the idea of 'unlocking the erotic fires that burn within', he didn't much fancy the prospect of unlocking the 'inner child'. He had heard about a prominent lawyer we know who was forced, during a recent workshop, to sit in a sandpit and talk to a gigantic teddy bear. The thought made him shudder.

But in the interests of my writing, he finally agreed to come with me. So we packed our sarongs, two pillows, and two towels and off we went. The course is part of a new world-wide movement called *Hot Monogamy*, aimed at saving the sacred institution of marriage.

With one in every two marriages breaking up, anyone who is anyone in the international relationships arena is searching for a solution to this growing problem. The latest wisdom is the concept of *Hot Monogamy* which focuses on keeping sex alive within long-term relationships.

There is a plethora of 'how-to' books hitting the streets as part of the movement. Videos like the Australian-made *Sacred Sex* and its sequels are doing a roaring trade around the world. Therapists are taking couples away on weekend retreats – all with the aim of ensuring couples continue to keep their relationships hot and spicy – and away from predators.

In Australia, several hotels are now cashing in on the trend of 'erotic time out' and are packaging dirty or romantic weekends away for married couples. I am told that some offer child-care on-site.

There are some very good courses available around the country through associations like The Pleasure Spot in Sydney and Human Awareness Australia based in Canberra. But the minute we arrived at this particular course, I knew it was a mistake.

The smell of incense was so strong we were almost bowled over. My husband suffers from hay fever and his inner child immediately started sneezing, much to the horror of our host who was trying to create a New Age ambience with whale music and shimmering candles.

We all stood around in a big circle rocking from side to side chanting some positive 'love mantra' whilst my poor darling sneezed and wheezed. The host finally banished him to a corner of the dimly lit room where he stood all hunched over and dejected, sniffing loudly to himself.

As the room slowly filled with billows of smoke, others

started to complain of suffocation. So the host eventually stormed off in a huff to put out his treasured incense.

After the 'group-bonding ritual' we were sent off with our partners to learn how to reconnect 'intimately'. We were given a tray of different enticements and told to experiment. There was fruit, silk scarves, ice cubes and a host of oils in bottles with different scents.

As instructed, I blindfolded my darling who had thankfully stopped sneezing. I then attempted to set his erotic energies on fire. I ran silk over his face and chest. He seemed to respond well. I fed strawberries into his little mouth. He giggled and laughed.

'Ask your partner how he or she likes to be touched,' the host urged. I was amused by this. After so long, wouldn't one know how one's partner liked to be touched? But my husband whispered something into my ear which really surprised me.

'Why have you never told me?' I said.

'Because you never asked,' he said.

He loved the feel of ice over his face and lips. We were suddenly in one of those erotic art films where people do strange, visceral things with egg yolks and bananas. As the music moaned its way to a crescendo I wanted to jump up and do erotic belly dancing and wild things with scarves. I felt my inner woman blend with my inner child. I felt untamed, passionate. As a final delight, I opened one of the little vials of oil and ran it under my husband's nose.

He was clearly in ecstasy, rolling his head from side to side in a euphoric frenzy. And then I realised something terrible. It wasn't a euphoric frenzy at all. It was a severe allergic reaction to the sacred aroma pong.

Sneezing, wheezing, coughing, spluttering followed. Gulping, snorting, honking, hooting. None of which was contributing to the general erotic ambience. In the interests of the group, we were asked to kindly continue lighting our erotic fires in our own home.

When he stopped sniffing and honking and we both stopped laughing we did indeed light our erotic fires. Because the truth is that *Hot Monogamy* – without the incense, whales and New Age mumbo jumbo – really has a lot going for it.

AFFAIRS

Anyone reading the papers recently would be forgiven for thinking that they're the only person in the entire country not having an affair.

Recently we saw another survey confirming that around 40 per cent of all Australians have had an extra curricular liaison. On radio we heard how women are now doing it more than men, and how at least 15 to 20 per cent of the population are serial adulterers. And to cap matters off, the chief censor, John Dickie, got in on the fracas saying that it was all due to the fact that we watched too many wicked movies about it.

Well, a big hello to all you wild adulterers out there. This is Ruth Ostrow calling. Come in, all you adulterers. Can you please tell my readers and I: How the hell do you guys find the time between the shopping and working, and meetings and children, to have an affair? And what are you eating for breakfast that gives you the energy?

Because I suspect we're all telling porkies again to feel potent. I don't know one person in my vast circle of friends who is really doing it. Don't get me wrong. We're not moralists. In fact, I surround myself with hedonists on principle. We all love the idea of copious, abundant, ceaseless nights of endless pleasure and passion. But the truth is, who has the time?

Sure we all fantasise about it. For me it goes something like this. I get a secret crush on someone – usually a dark, brooding type from a TV drama. At the moment it's Darcy from *Pride and Prejudice*. Darcy spots me out in viewer-land, sitting on the couch in my flannelette nightie and fluffy slippers. He must have me.

Out of the TV he jumps, compliments me on my awesome beauty, swoops me into his arms, removes my flannelette nightie with the duckies on the collar, ravishes my pulsating body, declares undying love then vanishes back into the TV set. The whole fantasy takes approximately 5 to 10 minutes. Usually during the commercial break, while my husband is off making a cup of tea.

Compare this, time wise, to the reality of an extramarital liaison.

You meet someone you fancy. The worrying begins. Does he want me? Will he ring? Worry, worry, love, goo, goo (wasted time: approximately 4 hours 30 minutes).

The first meeting. Probably over lunch or drinks. Awkward conversation. Trying to digest food. 'Blah, blah, blah,' giggle, pant, pant. Will he or won't he? (About 4 hours, including travel time).

Next day. Dreaming of him, love, love, moo, goo. Speak on phone. Set up meeting at hotel room. Worry, worry. Should we? Shouldn't we? Moo, goo, dream some more (Up to 5 hours).

The big night. Getting dressed. How do I look? Does my breath smell okay? Worry, worry. Excuses to partner. Lie, lie, lie. Get in car. Driving, driving (About 3 hours).

Arrive at hotel room. Stiff, awkward silence. Fumbling about. Clothes removed. Mouths collide. Things happen. Usually not great the first time. 'Sorry, sorry, I was too tense.'

Better luck next time. Wash, scrub, wash again. Drive home. Lie, lie, to partner. Get into bed. Worry. 'Can partner smell sex on me? Did lover think I was a disappointment?' Worry, worry, sleepless night (about 24 hours including recovery time).

Next day a bit itchy. A bit itchier. 'Oh God!' How do you ring someone and ask them if they've ever had genital warts? Herpes? Crabs? Snakes? Maybe it's the Ebola virus. 'Should have made him wear a condom!' Yell, yell at yourself inside your head. Ring doctor.

Drive to get blood test. 'What an idiot I am. I deserve to die.' Wait, wait, suffering. Terrible, awesome guilt. Hate lover. All their fault. Look at children. Guilt, guilt. Nightmares of broken home. Suffering, waiting. Get results. All clear. Just a case of Guilty Genitals (approximately 48 hours of total terror).

Phone rings. Lover wants reassurance. 'Was it good? Do you love me? You didn't just use me, did you?' Guilt, guilt. Terrible guilt. Lover wants to meet again. Deciding, thinking (about 45 minutes).

At this point at least you have wasted about 92 hours for a 10 second orgasm. It's like my mum always said about eating chocolate: 'A moment in the mouth, an eternity on the hips.'

Do you do it again? Apparently of those 40 per cent of people who reported this week that they had had an affair, 70 per cent said they would never do it again. Can you blame them?

All I can say is this. If almost half the married population can manage adultery between children, nappies, working, meetings with people, fighting with the plumber, paying the bills, and cleaning up, then my husband and I are changing our breakfast cereals.

HONEYMOON

We have finally done it, flown all the way to another city so that we can leave the baby with Mother for two days and have some time alone. Time alone, the concept has so profoundly escaped us over the past two years since she was born.

I can't even remember what it is like not to be glancing over my shoulder every moment to keep an eye on a very vibrant child. I can't remember what it feels like to lie in my husband's arms in bed at night without my ears pricked for any sign of a baby cry or snuffle.

The last time we were truly alone through the night without a baby in the next room, was on our honeymoon – just before she was born.

Alarming new statistics show that the minutes an average married couple spend alone, talking or touching intimately each week, can be counted on one hand. They also show that one in every two marriages is now ending in divorce.

I know from my readers' letters that those who set time aside for the relationship, for sex and love and indulgence, fare much better than those who neglect the small pleasures of life and who take each other for granted.

And so here we are. On a pilgrimage of pleasure. We have returned to the hotel where we spent the first night of our honeymoon to re-ignite the passion, and to spoil each other with languid love, to revel in *time out*.

The room is as it was then – all white and fluffy with lavishly draped curtains, a king-sized bed with extra large pillows and doona. We jump like crazed kids all over the bed, up and down, up and down. The sense of freedom is overwhelming.

We waste no time getting into the indulgence we came here for. I slip into one of those nice, fat, towelling robes that people used to steal before hotels caught on. My husband pops the cork on a bottle of French champagne, and we sit overlooking the city, guzzling down the bubbly and stuffing our faces with very rich, chocolate truffles from the mini bar.

As he runs a bath, I raid the mini bar again. Hotel mini bars are like Mount Everest. You raid them because they are there. I continue gorging myself on chips and cheese, nuts and pâté, and anything that looks remotely edible as we plan our 'pleasure itinerary' with all the fabulous and naughty things we are going to do over the next twenty-four hours.

It's a very tight schedule. At 6.30pm we intend to enter the black, marble bathroom and soak in the bubble bath until we feel totally euphoric. Downstairs by 8pm, for a wickedly expensive meal in the hotel restaurant. Then into bed by 10.30pm to catch the start of the adult video *Hot Love* advertised on the top of the television set. After that, passion until dawn and then breakfast in bed.

So many fantastic things to do now we are free...free... We're going to have great fun, and greater sex to really justify our time alone and, of course, the ludicrous cost of the hotel room.

Sitting in the very hot bubble bath I notice I am feeling a bit faint. I've eaten a few too many chips. I may have also jumped up and down on the bed too many times. The harsh jets of water pummelling my spine and feet and legs are not helping either. Sometimes spas can make you feel like you are being clubbed to death.

Then it begins. It starts in my temples and moves to the front of my head. The holiday headache. One of nature's cruelest jokes. You feel like a player who doesn't notice he's broken his leg until the game is over. When the pressure is off and it's time to relax, the brutal pain hits.

I swish two pain-killers down with a swig of champagne and we continue to plan our pleasure itinerary. But my husband is frowning. He has gone very red in the cheeks.

'I feel suddenly tired,' he says, stumbling out of the bath. 'Must have been the flight over and all that champagne. I'll just rest for a few moments,' he says. 'Then we can have some real fun.'

I get out of the bath too and flop beside him on the bed. We stare up at the ceiling feeling dreadful about feeling dreadful. The meter is ticking away. But it's hard work having a fabulous time on demand.

My darling puts his arm around me and we allow ourselves a brief cat-nap before dinner. We wake to the bell-desk ringing to ask us an odd question. Are we ready to check out?

My contact lenses are glued to my eyeballs. I stare in horror at the clock and the morning light. We bolt out of bed, dishevelled and guilty, and then we start laughing. Because it dawns on us. This is exactly what our wedding night was like, after all.

SLEEPING TOGETHER

I have never understood the presumption that because you enjoy having sex with someone, it automatically follows that you would want to sleep with them or rather sleep next to them – as in between the sheets, in the cot, and all that.

I was a great admirer of Harry in the film *When Harry Met Sally* who bravely volunteered that most men had a five-minute tolerance level for lolling about between the sheets after the great event.

Whilst five minutes of post-coital cuddling seems a bit frugal, at least we were hearing the words of an honest man. And honestly, when you think about it, there is no logical connection between wanting to wrap your body around another for

187

the purposes of carnal delight, and of thereafter wanting to have them glued to you like a rock-limpet for the next eight hours – certainly not every single time you do the business.

Even more to the point, there is no logical correlation between wanting to spend the rest of your life with someone in marital bliss and wanting to retreat to the same bedroom with them to sleep within inches of another writhing, squirming, possibly overheated and probably restless, human body every night of the week for the rest of your life.

Which is why in homes around Australia there is a steep increase in 'the other bedroom'.

I have been noticing this trend for a long time but only thought to write about it when I recently saw an article from an American magazine called 'Bed as a War Zone' based on a report that more and more couples were opting to keep separate sleeping quarters.

The reasons quoted included a sharp increase in male snoring. Already 20 per cent of males between the ages of thirty and thirty-five snore with this figure trebling for the over-sixties. There are now over a hundred anti-snoring devices registered with the US patent office, but separate sleeping is becoming one of the most popular ways of coping.

The article claims that twice as many women as men suffer from insomnia, prowling around the house, getting in and out of bed or shuffling restlessly till the break of dawn. This is driving a lot of men from the nuptial bed.

Given that it has always been common for aristocrats and royalty to have separate sleeping arrangements, it seems that the notion of sharing the nuptial bed came from necessity, probably because poorer families were forced to share sleeping quarters at various times throughout history.

But modern couples are now beginning to question this practice especially those with enough money to keep a spare bedroom or those whose high-pressured lives necessitate a good night's sleep.

However, despite the growing prevalence of separate sleeping, there is still a social stigma to admitting it. The couples I talked to for this article would not let themselves be named, as if there was some shame in not managing to spend an average of fifty-six hours a week on top of another human body.

Miraculously and most fortunately my husband and I do sleep well together, largely because he is a very heavy sleeper.

But I once lived with a man who used to wake me up every night with illogical babbling. I tried ear plugs but he would shake me awake, as if even in his sleep he needed an audience. Finally, one night, I retreated to the spare room in desperation.

This happy sleeping arrangement continued till we finally split. It suited us both because he also hated me reading in bed. The sound of flipping pages had really annoyed him.

One couple jokes that they are lucky enough to have a house big enough to have a spare room. 'It's a luxury not always having to sleep together,' she chortles. 'An investment in our future,' says her partner. The problem for this couple is different time clocks. She loves to sit up late watching schlock TV and would drive him nuts shuffling about when she finally came to bed. He would bother her early in the morning opening and shutting drawers.

One woman who usually sleeps separately from her spouse reckons that she used to hit him in her sleep. Apparently this is quite a common occurrence like sleep-walking. During sleep many subconscious aggressions come out which is healthy for the dreamer, but not so good for those sleeping nearby.

My husband has just read over this, and wants to say that he is not at all happy with the temperature of our bed. He claims it is like an oven with my electric blanket radiating enough heat to cook a chicken. He says that if we had a spare room he'd sleep in there with the windows wide open so he could bask in the frosty night air.

Interestingly, in my discussions with people, different body temperatures rated highly as a force driving people from the same bed, alongside doona stealing, teeth grinding, and thrashing about. But those sleeping separately should take heart. If it's good enough for royalty, then surely it's good enough for us common folk.

STRIP TEASE

I am poncing around the lounge room shaking my love-'thang' at my husband. 'My darling I…can't get enough of your love, babe.' I croon, singing Barry White. My husband is not watching. He is far more interested in the John Howard item on the news.

In case he hasn't got the message, I throw my shoes in his direction, and keep dancing about…'I don't know, I don't know why…can't get enough of your love…babe.'

Still no response. Men who are married to women with small children, do not expect any love-thang to be shaken at them after about 10.30 at night. And they certainly stop shaking their love-thang at you.

Can't blame them really. It must be very demoralising to stare romantically into the tired, hollow eyes of a woman who has spent the day trailing around after a toddler. Or worse. A woman who has spent the day at the office and the evening trailing around after a toddler. 'Hello in there? Hello?' Lights on, nobody home!

But I've got something very special in store tonight. 'Ohhh babe...' I drawl and throw my top at him. It hits his face. He keeps watching TV oblivious of my love dance. He doesn't realise that I have not really been out all evening with my girl-friends. I lied. I went instead to a class given by one of Australia's best known strip-tease artists Elizabeth Burton.

Having written so copiously about the dangers of letting marriages fall into boring, non-erotic spaces, I reckoned I had to find a way to inject a bit of spice around the house. I think it was the letters that terrified me.

Bags of mail from people who talked about how sex took a complete and utter nose-dive after children came along. The US statistics someone sent me warned that one child takes a huge chunk out of your libido. Two is worse than one, and God help anyone with three kids or more.

Meanwhile men grizzled bitterly that their wives never bothered to wear sexy lingerie. One whined his wife wore so many layers of flannelette it took ten minutes to get it all off, by which time he had lost his motivation. Others grumbled that the onus was still very much on men to instigate sex, and create atmosphere.

So off I went to join a group of raunchy and courageous women, many with small children at home, who don't want to let their marriages or relationships go into decline. These babes, in all shapes and sizes, are committed to remaining erotic.

The strip-tease courses are run regularly by Jo-Anne Baker of The Pleasure Spot in Sydney. But they are not the only spicy courses women, men or couples can do to put a bit of zing back into domestic life. Her course, which she runs around the country, includes Tantra and Eastern lovemaking techniques, erotic massage, belly dancing, erotic photography.

'Relationships don't have to go stale,' says Baker, whose cheeks light up a glowing red as the music starts thudding out White's cry of love: 'Can't get enough of your love, babe...'

Our teacher Elizabeth, a leggy blonde in bikini and stilettos, puts her hands to her hair and starts mincing around the room. 'I want you ladies to start strutting. Feel the beauty of your bodies,' she says as the music tempo starts to rise.

'Your own body is beautiful no matter what shape.'

Women being women do not believe a word of it. We all stand about looking tense and doubtful and we are praying we won't have to remove too many items of our day-wear.

'Any man should be thrilled you are doing this for him. Believe you are lovely,' and with this she suddenly throws off her clothes and stands there in the nuddy, 'just to show that my body isn't perfect, either.' She is close to fifty and close enough to perfect. But she is making a very important point.

If you believe yourself sexy, you will look sexy because you will exude a lovely confidence and sensuality.

There is such magic in being a woman. Such a joyous sexual energy that we are taught to repress. As career women, any hint of sexuality is now an act of incitement to sexual harassment. As mothers we feel guilty about expressing it because sensuality and motherhood don't go together in many women's heads.

But here, in this room, we can all rejoice the business of being female and suddenly the room is alive as socks go flying across the room. Smelly shoes are coming off, and old shirts are flying into space. There is a buzz and excitement that is intoxicating. We're becoming feral. Back to our wild primordial roots. 'Can't get enough... Ooooh babe... can't get enough...'

Back at home my husband finally realises I mean business.

He takes his eyes off the TV and his mouth falls to the floor as he realises I still have a love-thang. It certainly pays to try something a little wild and wonderful sometimes. Demi Moore eat your heart out!

FLIRTING

I recently caught my husband flirting with another woman.

We were at a party. I had wandered off to get a drink and before I'd taken ten steps some babe, all curls and smiles, had moved in for the kill. Given the chronic shortage of straight, available male talent in this country, it doesn't take too long these days for a man standing alone at a party to be supper.

From where I was standing I saw the sudden change in his posture and I particularly noticed the change in body language.

The experts say to look for feet pointed towards the love interest. I could swear, even at that distance, that my husband's foot was pointing not only towards the woman but directly up at her private parts. What's worse he was moving that foot around every which way like some deranged magnet searching for the right direction. She obliged by subconsciously moving her legs apart.

After a few moments she began playing with her hair which is a sign of intimacy. Then she leaned forward, smiling and baring her teeth – the ultimate show of animal attraction. I knew under her clothing her bottom was probably turning red like those mating baboons on nature programs.

Anyway I remained at a distance observing the game. He was clearly having a wonderful time. I presumed from the way he was puffing his chest out that he was telling the fire story – the one about the time he leapt to the defence of our apartment block by single-handedly putting out a raging fire.

She was gazing adoringly at this urban hero whose other feats include being able to open a sealed glass pickled-cucumber jar with a single swoop, and who – when our lawn-mower was broken – spent several Saturdays manually lopping off every blade of grass with a pair of scissors. Though some would have recommended psychiatric treatment, my husband to this day remains very proud of this great achievement.

Anyway I was prepared to be all jealous and angry but as I watched the interaction it occurred to me how mandatory the whole act of flirting really was in modern life.

It was clearly important for my husband to be reasserting his manhood. What pleasure it was giving him recounting the fire story and beating his breast like some primitive beast.

Poor men are still being socialised by films that equate maleness with heroism – saving aircraft from terrorist hijacks, saving the planet from nuclear destruction. On film real men 'boldly go where no man has gone before'. In reality most end up in the suburbs fretting that there are no damsels to save or universes to rescue.

When they do manage some basic act of heroism like saving a dog from being run over or working out how to pre-program the video recorder, their partners barely offer a patronising smile.

Men desperately need babes with open mouths and dilated pupils to show off to, to brag about work achievements to, to get an ego hit from. It's a basic, primordial need that harks back to male animals trying to impress females and implant their seed.

So here was my husband subconsciously sussing out the seed planting potential and clearly loving every delicious minute of it. But the exercise was equally important for me. If one puts aside the apprehension that one is going to be abandoned, rejected, betrayed, and just allows flirting to be what it is, there is a wonderful resonance to it.

Much as we may love our partners, it is easy to take someone you live with for granted. But when you see your partner through the adoring eyes of another, passion flares up and you remember what it was that won you over. A little animal jealousy goes a long way.

I might add, the female species also needs to show off their coloured bits occasionally. And I think our partners also like to see us flashing our coloured bits at other males. It arouses the competitive spirit and gets the testosterone flowing.

Anyway after this party my husband and I went home and had a very hot time, and I really have to ask: what is so wrong with sexual energy being created from sources other than ourselves? Why are we so hung up on being the only source of our partner's turn-on? Why are women in particular so jealous when their partners flirt?

In many countries of Europe it is quite natural for both men and women to relate to the world sexually. Flirting is a natural turn-on, as is watching the opposite sex from the sidewalk coffee shops.

As long as you bring the sexual excitement you are feeling home, then what is wrong with admiring others, fantasising about others or experiencing the joy of watching them get turned on by you? The answer is, nothing.

When done from the safety of a secure marriage I think flirting can be one of the most erotic, pleasurable things to do and probably more likely to prevent cheating than create it.

EROTICA

It sounds like a scene from some erotic movie. A couple staring deep into each other's eyes as they share their most secret, sexual fantasies. But it is not a scene in a movie, rather it is really happening out in the suburbs of Victoria.

Still on my search for solutions to keeping marriages hot, I go to see Professor Marita McCabe at the Deakin University psychology department. After finding that at least 30 per cent of people in long-term relationships were sexually dissatisfied with their partners, she has set up a sexual fantasy therapy program at a clinic run by the university, to help couples deal with the problem of flagging sex-lives.

The program, which is designed to teach people how to use sexual fantasy to put the zing back into their marriages, is the first of its kind in Australia and is still highly experimental. Professor McCabe believes that the happiest marriages and relationships are those where the erotic side is very much alive.

She says problems for couples often begin because one person wants more sex than the other can provide. She says it is becoming more common for women to discover sex as they get older, which is when most men are coming off the boil. As this problem gets more acute, men will often avoid sex to avoid confronting their flagging libidos. Because her research has shown that men tend to control frequency of sex in marriage, shifts in libido can be disastrous for a lot of couples.

Professor McCabe feels that sexual fantasy and erotic thought often help men retain erections during their later years, and help bring sex back into the marriage. She says men are highly visual and can be easily stimulated. Fantasy can give men back their confidence. But sadly, many women feel threatened by their husband's psychological infidelities.

'We're trying to teach women that jealousy and anxiety often impede sexuality. If women allow themselves to engage in erotica it would help men and it would enhance their sex-lives.

'We're also trying to teach both men and women how to fantasise. Many people won't give themselves permission to think erotic thoughts, because they feel it means they are kinky or weird or that they are going to go out and do the thing they are fantasising about.

'Often the reverse is true. The fantasy is the opposite of what a person would really do in real life. It is healthy to fantasise and it can create real intimacy between couples if they share their thoughts and feelings.'

She says that while men experience frequency problems later in life, women can have the same problems after children are born. 'They start seeing themselves as mothers, and the concept of mother is not a sexual one for most people.'

Professor McCabe says she starts the program by getting couples to listen to erotic tapes of Anais Nin stories. Then she tries to unlock their visual powers by encouraging them to go out and buy some erotic magazines or watch erotic movies. She says women get excited by visual stimulation, too.

'We get couples pleasuring each other. After they become more visual and graphic we get them into sensuality and touch. Then we get them flirting with each other by encouraging them to remember all the positive things that brought them together.'

She says if people stopped feeling threatened by jealousy, then all the sexual energy that erotica created could be channelled back into the relationship to inspire lust. She says it pays to remember the adage: 'It doesn't matter where you get your appetite, as long as you eat at home.'

MASTER OF THE HOUSE

I have never understood my mother's attitudes to sex, nor she mine. It has always been like two islands with no bridge in the middle. She, coming from England and a culture that valued reticence and reserve above all else. Me, growing up in Australia in an era of mass communication, of women's liberation, of Germaine Greer and Erica Jong sharing their affairs in graphic, gynaecological detail with the whole world.

'Is nothing private to you?' my mother has asked repeatedly over the years as I've launched from sexploit to sexploit with glee, and compounded the sin by writing about it all. 'No,' I have said to her and continue to say. 'No, I don't do anything that the rest of the world isn't doing daily. So why is it private?'

But last week someone kindly sent me some photocopied pages of a textbook apparently distributed to schools throughout Australia and New Zealand in the '50s for the subject then known as Home Economics. I laughed heartily when I read it, and suddenly it was as if a bridge appeared out of the fog.

A bridge not only linking me to my mother and her values but to many of my older readers who write to me each week confused and affronted by my open and permissive attitudes to sexuality and relationships.

Not forty years ago women were being taught officially, through the education system, the sorts of lessons that today's modern women cannot in our wildest imaginations fathom.

The chapter 'How To Be A Good Wife' begins thus: 'When he comes home from work, listen to him. You may have a dozen important things to tell him, but the moment of his arrival is not the time. Let him talk first, remember, his topics of conversation are more important than yours.

'Have dinner ready. Prepare yourself. Touch up your

make-up, put a ribbon in your hair and be fresh looking. He has just been with a lot of work weary people. His boring day may need a lift and one of your duties is to provide it. Clear away the clutter. Gather up school books, toys and papers. Then run a dust cloth over the tables.

'Prepare the children. Take a few minutes to wash the children's hands and faces, comb their hair and if necessary change their clothes. They are little treasures and he would like to see them playing the part.

'Minimise all noise. Try to encourage the children to be quiet. Greet him with a warm smile and show sincerity in your desire to please and serve him.'

My favourite lesson for aspiring wives concerns sex: 'Never complain if he comes home late or goes out to dinner or other places of entertainment without you. Don't complain, even if he stays out all night. Count this as minor compared to what he went through during his day.'

A similar book on the subject implies that wives would probably count it as a blessing if their husbands stayed out all night: 'After coitus, the husband must allow the wife to repair to the bathroom. He must not go after her for she will want to shed a few tears.' Such is her suggested abhorrence to the act.

The lesson concludes: 'Don't ever ask him about his actions or question his integrity. Remember he is the *master* of the house and as such will exercise his will with fairness and truthfulness. You have no right to question him. A good wife will always know her place.'

I read this out to my husband as he carries the shopping bags into the kitchen and walks around unpacking them and chasing the baby around the room to stop her writing on the walls with her new crayons. He laughs loudly and laments that he was not born into a time when man was truly king.

But when I read it to my mother, there is no laughter. 'This is exactly how it was for me,' she sighs. 'You children were always washed and clean the moment before your father came home. You were kept quiet. I was always made-up, with dinner waiting. He came home and read the paper in silence. I can't believe you don't remember how it was,' she says growing close to tears.

I don't remember. I remember only the '70s and the excited whispers as women began congregating around tables discussing Greer and the feminist books they were reading. I remember the tones of elation and joy as women realised that they were not born to serve, and the delight when they realised their bodies were indeed capable of great pleasure.

But not all women realised. And having now seen these textbooks, I am amazed – not that the open discussion of sexuality and relationships has elicited such an angry response in some of my older readers, but that more people are not angrier: women because their generation was denied this wonderful sexual freedom, and men because women like me came along and spoiled the party.

CABIN FEVER

Do you ever inexplicably feel the urge to stab your beloved in the arm with a blunt toothbrush? Do you suddenly feel like pouncing on the one you love and bludgeoning them on the head with a pillow or squeegee?

Relax. Chances are you are not falling out of love. Chances are that you are just temporarily spatially challenged. By spatially challenged I do not mean 'a short person or midget' as politically correct lingo would have it put.

I mean you are feeling spatially cramped, hemmed in, choked, stifled, stymied, suffocated. 'I need space,' you scream inside your head but no-one, least of all your partner and brood of kids, is listening.

The mere sight of your partner makes you want to throw yourself headlong off a cliff. When he or she smiles you feel the urge to set the house alight with gelignite. Especially if it is one of those ingratiating 'What have I done wrong?' sort of smiles that make you feel guilty for wanting to perform wanton acts of barbarism.

You want to yell: 'Nothing is wrong with you. It's me. It's me. I hate you because you exist. Because every time I come into a room you are there smiling at me.'

Now whilst politically correct people will be undoubtedly distressed by the level of violence expressed here, I doubt anyone living with another human being in a full-time, full-on, relentless and irreversible state of permanence will not understand what I am saying.

It's cabin fever – an old American term that was used to describe the deranged behaviour exhibited by people trapped in their cabins for weeks during snowstorms. Now used to describe the hysteria and panic people feel after spending too long on an international flight. Synonym: Stir crazy. It is a well-established fact that people in marriages or long-term, live-in situations can go as stir crazy as prisoners in a Turkish jail. In fact, after a few years of marriage, many would opt for a Turkish jail – with the torture thrown in.

Cabin fever has traditionally been the emotional terrain of males. I have always believed men invented war, territorial conflict and bloody religious altercations so they could put on their heavy armour and march away for years at a time, to get away from their smiling female permanent others.

Then when war became unfashionable, they began building businesses and invading corporations so they could stay too busy to come home to their crammed caves. The money helped buy bigger caves so the wife and children could be further away. But not far enough. Never far enough. So they built sheds in their backyards and walled off *home offices* for themselves, to make escape easier.

Now women have caught the dreaded disease. With the multitude of stressful roles we must now play in the wake of economic equality, it is impossible not to feel overcome, exhausted, trapped, and hemmed in.

The problem with trendy role sharing is that men are at home more doing the ironing, shopping and child minding. In fact, everyone is at home. Aaarrch! I am told that when husbands first retire, stir crazy wives will often lunge at them with kitchen appliances or try to iron their faces.

Anyway, with husband and I both working from home, I got a bad case of cabin fever a few weeks ago. At first I didn't know what it was. In all our years of living together, I had never felt anything quite as passionate.

I found myself staring at my husband's socks and wanting to set them on fire. I felt totally invaded by the bits of paper and coffee mugs he had spread over my desk.

'You two should go out to dinner together,' my well-meaning mother suggested. 'For a romantic evening.' I ran and hid the wallet.

Finally a friend stepped in. 'You just need a holiday from each other. A bit of space. It's hard being together all the time, and having a toddler to boot. It's only natural you're going stir crazy.'

This made sense. I tried to tell my husband as delicately as I could that I needed a break. He looked very hurt. I was about to cancel my arrangements when I heard him talking to a mutual friend on the phone.

'Ruth is going away,' he was almost singing into the mouthpiece. 'I feel delighted. Overjoyed!'

The thing that I realised about cabin fever is that it is highly contagious. For the first few days your partner doesn't know how to appease you. Then he or she begins to resent your bad moods, which makes you resent their bad moods about your bad moods. 'Hey, whose bad mood is this anyway?'

The next day I left for a short break. At first, I didn't think of home at all. The second day I was tempted to ring, but I overcame the urge. The third day I was curious and called home actually happy to hear my partner's voice. By day four I had rung three times, and by day five I was running off the train into his arms with excited glee.

We rushed back to our cabin, locked the door and whilst baby was at mother-in-law's bolted ourselves in for hours. Funny, even with the doors and windows locked, the air was suddenly fresh and crisp and invigorating.

DOING DEALS

I would once again like to take up an issue that has proved enormously controversial with my readers – paying partners for sex.

A couple of months ago I ran this genuine letter from a woman in Victoria. 'In the shower after squash at my local centre some of the women talk about how much they charge their husbands for sex. Some claim they charge $80 a time. The wife of a doctor even claims she gives her husband a heavy smack on the bum whenever he doesn't produce money before the act. They tell me I should do the same to my fiancé, especially after we get married. Do many women charge their husbands or boyfriends for sex? How much is an appropriate sum?'

A letter the following week stirred up even more trouble than the first. A woman from Gawler in South Australia wrote: 'If a husband is prepared to pay a prostitute to have either straight sex or something kinky, then wouldn't it be better to pay that to his wife for his requests? It certainly helps the family budget.'

What followed was nothing short of outrage. Pamela from Brisbane snorted that the women were nothing but 'gold diggers'. 'It is better not to be married at all if you see your partner as a client, not as someone you love,' she wrote.

But the worst anger came from men. 'Your friends are fools and if there are more women in the world out there like them, us males should stay single. Love does not cost anything, why should sex?' grumbled R.J., of Toowoomba in Queensland.

'Disgusted Male' wrote: 'I know the average woman is still "carried" financially [by men] on a free ride through life. But to learn they brag about selling sex to husbands or partners is tragic. Male victims world-wide still empty smelly garbage, fix flat tyres, lift heavy equipment, but sex will always be a transaction.'

Mr 'J' from Lidcombe in New South Wales wrote: 'If "Anon" is going to charge for sex after marriage, it is hoped that she will provide variety and value for money and not expect her husband to settle for the usual "dead fish" performance rendered by most wives. I wonder how women would react if husbands insisted on payment for the suffering they endure through the senseless, never-ending, boring, chatter inflicted on them by their partners who consider themselves to be engaging in interesting and meaningful discussions.'

I got a lot of letters from both males and females who were angry at the tired old myth that for women sex in marriage was a chore. Alan of Annerley in Queensland surprised me with this one: 'I work in a Therapeutic Massage centre and am amazed by the number of women who phone up looking for sex and not just sex, but kinky sex. Men are not the only ones who enjoy sex, so let these women stop playing the martyr and making out they are doing their husbands a favour. Let's hear it for equality and let the men charge their wives for sex.'

Meanwhile Barry of Adelaide cheerfully wrote: 'Female friends have told me how pathetic most guys are at making love. I am still laughing at the average times of two to ten minutes from your last article. So I say, ladies, make him pay in dollars if your guy isn't good enough to make you want to pay him.'

One of the saddest letters came from 'D' in Burleigh, Queensland: 'My wife actually pays me *not* to have sex. After the first year of marriage she completely lost her libido. She couldn't wait to get finished and carry on with the ironing. She didn't like the way her attitude was hurting me so she suggested that whenever I felt a bit randy, she would give me a few dollars to go down to the pub for a few beers. By the time I got back, she would be already asleep. Now I am fast becoming an alcoholic! What should I do?'

A couple of years ago I stayed with friends who had a wonderful solution to the problem of sex, money and power, in a long-term relationship. It was a very equitable proposal and one my readers may wish to consider.

My girlfriend and her partner kept a little notebook much

like the exercise books we had in school. Each time one of them did something good or meritorious, they were awarded gold stars. Each star counted for one dollar. Different deeds earned different points. For instance, washing the dishes may win five stars, taking the children out to the park might earn ten.

The notebook was like a bank, and when either of my friends had accumulated enough gold stars, they could ask their partner to buy them something that correlated with the dollar value they had accrued. It could be a cassette or a new jumper, depending on the amount of stars in their book.

But at some point in time the game turned very erotic. Charging market rates, they began trading their stars for sexual favours.

Delicacy prevents me from going into detail, but I can only confirm that the two of them were always busy doing good deeds. They were the goodest deed doers I had ever seen, falling over each other to do the dishes, cook the dinner, wash the clothes, communicate their 'deepest' feelings, and baby-sit.

My husband and I tried the system following our stay and I can honestly report that it was the most erotically charged summer we had ever spent together. Sadly, as with all things, life got in the way and we let the system lapse.

But it seems to be a system that not only keeps sex fun, cheeky and naughty, it also keeps the house in order, and the relationship thriving with interesting conversation. In fact, I think we just may have stumbled on the ideal solution to the problem of *Hot Monogamy*.

LETTERS

Dear Ruth,

You wanted our tips for how to keep our marriage hot. Here they are: my husband and I put aside at least one night a week to turn the lights down low, turn off the television (one of the greatest modern disasters for a healthy sex-life!) and get into some deep reconnecting. It's amazing how sexy old-fashioned intimacy can be.

D.A., ST KILDA, VIC

Dear Ruth,

This is the reason that affairs begin. The desire for excitement, passion, intimacy, all of which seems to get lost along the way for many women in the early years of family raising. The first affair was electric. The tenth will be my last, but by no means my least. My husband knows nothing of them; my marriage of thirty-five years is looked upon by my friends as being an ideally suited couple. I don't think we would be together now had I not had real life 'fantasies'. So, Ruth, believe it!

ANON., SYDNEY, NSW

Dear Ruth,

I think you are a disgusting woman writing as you do, really encouraging people to be unfaithful. Do you ever stop to think of the broken homes that occur through having affairs and the sadness to wives who love their husbands and to the children of these families? It has many times caused terrible suffering, even death on many occasions. Some men have also suffered deeply.

D.F., CLARENCE GARDENS, SA

HOT & SWEATY

Dear Ruth,

Thank you for revealing to others that sleeping in separate rooms does not mean the end of your sex-life. I have been in my own room for two years, after twenty 'sleep disturbed' years with a hundred-decibel snorer. Now there is bliss on both sides. Peace for me after my 'visits', and no more broken ribs for him!

BEST THING, ELANORA, QLD

Dear Ruth,

Thank God, I'm normal. I'm thirty-nine, happily married sixteen years with two wonderful children. I want to change to single beds. I'm sick of being breathed on with beer smelling breath, being kicked with knees and having covers taken.

ANNE, BUDERIM, QLD

Dear Ms Ostrow,

As a married mother of a two-year-old toddler, I want to say that after a hard day at work or home all I want is a nice quiet place to retreat to on my own. Sex has become a weekly event like putting out the garbage. While my partner and I are unhappy about this development, thank God we are not part of the 10 per cent of couples who *never* do it at all.

DEBBIE C., BRONTE, NSW

Dear Ruth,

You don't have to be single to be lonely. I'm married and have four children, three still at home, and I am so lonely that I sit and cry for hours. I'm in a loveless marriage. Why do people think just because you're married and have a family you can't get lonely?

MRS S., HIGHPOINT CITY, VIC

CHAPTER SIX

HOT & SWEATY UNDER THE COVERS:
What really turns us on

GIVEN that I spend a large portion of my time writing about and pondering on matters sexual, my readers could be forgiven for thinking that I lead a rather exotic life. I too was under this delusion until a little book arrived on my desk which forced me to re-evaluate things.

After spending a few hours reading through *The Planet Sex Handbook*, I can only conclude that in fact I lead a most parochial and sheltered life. Indeed, after reading this, I may even add the word 'dull'.

The handbook is published in England by the reputable sexpert Tuppy Owens, author of the infamous *Sex Maniac's Diary* and organiser of the equally infamous Sex Maniac's Ball which she holds in London each year to raise money for charity.

Apparently, high society patrons and matrons pay vast sums of money to attend the annual event which includes an 'under the table' service with volunteer sex maniacs crawling around the floor pleasuring guests while they eat.

Anyway, Owens, who has a degree in Human Sexuality from London University, is a girl after my own heart. She has spent years travelling around the world researching all the various clubs and associations people frequent in order to indulge their sexual passions. She has collated this bizarre information of what turns people on into *The Planet Sex Handbook*.

So what does turn people on? The first eye-opener came when I read under the 'H' listing that there are clubs world-wide for lovers of hairy women. There is a club called Daughters of Hirsutism in Chicago and a publication called *Hair Apparent* for those who like their females unshaved and *au naturel*.

If this makes you squirm you may want to join The Smoothie Club in the UK for 'people who like shaved, smooth bodies'. The US club is called Bushwackers. One can only speculate as to why.

There are people who get turned on wearing raincoats. They would be well-advised to join a club called International Mackintosh Society in the UK. Owens says they 'put on annual weekends, and events abroad'. Very jolly indeed, but don't forget to pack your raincoat.

There are clubs for people who get their rocks off wearing all manner of things but I think the one that shocked me most was under 'A' for adult babies. Precious Baby Wear in England, and Especially For Me in California apparently supply super-sized diapers, bibs, dummies and other paraphernalia. Once dressed, adult babies can go to various playgroups in these cities. Both Diaper Pail Friends, and Mummy Hazel's Hush-a-bye Baby Club, offer special events in playpens with nursemaids. All I can say is the nurses must have very strong arms.

I was amused by a listing for a wonderfully strange group of people called Giantess Lovers. According to Owens they are: 'people who want to be trampled'.

There is a fellow who frequents Sydney's fantasy house, Club Medea, and gets turned on pretending he is a doormat. In summer he goes to the beach, burrows into the sand and puts his towel on top so that people will unwittingly frolic over him.

For those who find this story unbelievable there are several associations around the world that cater to this very obsession. Mr Carpet is based in Pocono Summit USA and is presumably a place where other carpets can meet and have a good time. There is Giantess in New York selling 'books and magazines on gigantic women with enormous boobs crushing and interacting with wimps'. There is also Squish in California for people who 'dream of big barefoot ladies trampling them'.

The Hung Jury is a club in Los Angeles for men with giant penises and the women who love them. Meanwhile Taloned Women is a newsletter for those who get turned on by 'women with long nails and scratching'. Australians can join a number of swingers' groups or join a club for lovers of fishnet stockings or pop over to a club in Japan for men who want to do weird things with fish.

Under the chapter 'Shopping' Owens gives a big thumbs-up to Fetters: 'A wonderful group of friendly people who make bondage and fetish wear caringly and with empathy'. She also likes Eroteak in the UK whose 'hand-made dungeon and sexy furniture has now reached amazing standards'.

Those away from home may benefit from Ms Owens' helpful translations. She teaches her readers to say: 'My wife and I would like to make it with you,' in German, Arabic or Welsh. Meanwhile you can say: 'I am a masochist. I need a sadist,' in

Portuguese, and even Hebrew for those looking for action in the Holy City.

Anyway, following in the footsteps of the marvellously entertaining Owens, I turn my attentions in this chapter to the alluring question of what really turns us on. What really goes on under the covers?

I take up where Owens leaves off, having spent the past year hanging about in dungeons, visiting sex-clubs, road-testing sex-toys and interviewing the weirdest and wildest people, in a bid to bring you a shockingly intimate portrait of the world after dark.

For your sakes, I have peeped into people's windows, into their hearts and ultimately into their bedrooms. May this chapter make you *hot and sweaty* all over.

'MERCY, MISTRESS'

Mistress Medea is exhausted. She has had a really busy week. She has organised a slave auction which will be held in the next few weeks. She has been putting the final touches on the dungeons she rents out to couples for the special rate of $75 an hour. And she's been running mistress training workshops to help her staff get into shape.

All this while attending to the regular day-to-day duties of running her new S&M haunt, Club Medea – Australia's first private S&M club. It is 2am and Medea has just finished disciplining a prominent QC in the schoolroom upstairs when I go to see her.

'It's pretty tiring,' she says, leaning back in a chair and dragging passionately at a cigarette. She is one of the most extraordinary-looking women I have ever seen. Tall, with a magnificent body and long, black hair, she looks every bit the male fantasy. Tonight she is wearing a provocative black catsuit of transparent mesh. Her nipples are huge and visible. I try to keep my eyes above the neck, but it's hard to concentrate.

'As soon as we opened the door we were swamped by requests for membership,' she says, oblivious to my breast envy. 'We already have 500 people on our books and there are new inquiries every day.

'But I love this work. It's the best job I've had.'

Medea's former work included many years as a finance journalist under the name Sandra Van Dijk and then press secretary to a well-known government minister. We chat about my years as a finance journalist and share private stories about 'in-depth interviews' we conducted. Basically concurring that businessmen are indeed a kinky breed of the human species.

In fact, she says it was during her years of interviewing, and working with leading businessmen, lawyers and politicians that she realised what a huge demand for her current services there was at the upper echelons of society.

'At $300 an hour, and up to $500 for *special* requests, it is a rich man's sport,' she says. 'We get some of the most prominent people in Australia through here each night – women as well as men.' The fee does not include traditional sex. 'Nothing as boring as that,' she grins mysteriously.

Medea's lover, a Sydney businessman, helped her set up the club which is run from a three-storey Victorian terrace in Sydney's inner city and is lavishly decked out in rich black and red fabrics. But she doesn't want to give too much away about him. 'He is fairly well-known in the finance world, and his child goes to a private school, so I have to be sensitive,' she says.

She says her clients pay for a qualified mistress or master to play out their fantasies, whether it be to get spanked, or to take them back to their school days. 'S&M is intellectual sex. It is about using the mind.'

She says that while many of her clients are wealthy or famous, she is trying to make the club accessible to the mainstream by hiring out dungeons to couples. 'The couples that come here often want to just indulge in some light, erotic play. We get plenty of your garden-variety, people-next-door coming along each night.'

She says she opened Medea's because: 'I get a lot of pleasure from this work.' Pleasure is a not a word that comes readily to mind, touring the dungeons and fantasy rooms of the house.

The dungeons are equipped with racks, and various instruments of torture. In one, a naked woman is being whipped by a near-naked mistress in a military hat. Medea says the woman comes to the club twice a week. A third of Medea's members are female.

A door accidentally catches the wind as we pass and opens just enough for me to catch a glimpse of a woman in a nurse's uniform standing open legged above a naked male who is lying on a mattress on the floor. In her hand is a strap-on dildo.

Quickly and aggressively she slams the door shut. There are sudden murmurs from two other mistresses who have seen what happened. They come rushing up and ask me if I recognised the man. I assure them I am myopic and they remind me that I am not to write anything without Medea's approval. 'We get a lot of very high-profile people in here. Their confidentiality must be respected.'

At that point I hear someone else yell, 'He's here.' And I am bundled into a side room with the door shut until 'he' passes. It is clear from the tension in the air that this is one of those well-known men who I am told are usually celebrities or people in high-profile, high-pressure positions. The coast is clear and we are back on our way.

The medical room has a doctor's table along with sutures and, can it be? Injections. The schoolroom has desks, teddies, blackboard. And of course an extra large ruler for teacher to use on aberrant children. There are any number of vibrators and phalluses around the joint, of varying sizes. Man size, snack size and bite size.

Mistress Medea smiles at my naivety. 'Pleasure is what it is all about. Pleasure and pain are inextricably linked,' she says citing her own exhilaration at a recent bellybutton piercing she had done. 'I sort of went out of my body. You release certain chemicals when you are in pain and it makes you feel high.'

But most people get no pleasure in going to the dentist, childbirth, even getting one's legs waxed. Again she smiles. 'The pain has to be associated with sexual pleasure. Not just pain on its own. It's the combination that is so potent for my clients – and for me.' She hands me what looks like a black leather bikini and urges me to experiment.

It takes quite a bit of convincing but finally I put on the garment, and allow myself to be harnessed in a dog's collar and led downstairs to the dungeon. Medea tells me she wants to let me spend a bit of time in the cage, so I can contemplate my bad behaviour.

I sit alone in the cage for about twenty minutes. Out of boredom I calculate that at close to $5 a minute this is a very expensive form of foreplay for the businessmen and celebrities who come here. Especially considering that you could be thrown in jail overnight for free, and there'd be a meal or two included. I wonder if the clients think it's good value.

Medea pops in for a moment to ask if I'm okay, which I

think is very nice under the circumstances. Being an honest woman I admit that I'd like the little blow-heater in the corner to be turned on because it is very draughty on the floor and I suffer from the cold. It seems very odd to be telling a mistress about my bad circulation from the confines of a cage in a dungeon, but she cheerfully obliges.

When she returns she is not as cheerful. She has become firm and disciplinarian. She unlocks the cage and ties me up to a black leather chair and bosses me around. I hate being bossed around. I start to feel nervous. Then she picks up what looks like a horsewhip and I almost pass out. The things writers will do to provide atmosphere.

She tells me that if at any time I want her to stop, all I have to do is beg for mercy. She says the idea that you lose all control is one of the many misconceptions about S&M. 'What people don't understand is that there are firm rules to this game. The slave and dominatrix have mutual respect for each other. A slave only has to say "Mercy, Mistress" and all pain stops. Our clients tell us what they want or can tolerate before the ritual begins. S&M is about safe sex in every way.'

I feel immediately relieved and ready for the punishment I must endure. But after a few lashes I start feeling wimpy. I have always been averse to smacking or hitting since my sister walloped me with a thong when I was young. I remember clearly the sting as the rubber object of torture descended on my nubile thigh. I sat in the corner and screeched until my mother scooped me up and calmed me down. Thereafter all thongs were banned from our house.

And now, instead of any erotic inspirations, with each flay all I can think about is a pair of over-sized, blue, rubber thongs. Which makes me think of men with fat feet walking along the beach in summer and mothers in thongs screaming after their screaming kids who are wearing thongs...

The mind is free-falling. Hidden associations are coming thick and fast with every lash just as Medea promised. These are my deepest, darkest thoughts. And they are horrible. Thongs. More thongs. More fat feet in thongs...walking along the pavement...standing at barbecues...'Mercy, Mistress!' I yell.

'I have a low pain threshold,' I mutter in embarrassment as she unties me.

'Ummmm thanks,' I say on the way out of the dungeons. I don't know if it is S&M etiquette to thank your persecutor but I've been brought up to be polite. On the way out we pass a whole lot of metal objects. 'Branders,' she says, 'like the ones used for branding cattle. Often we use them on slaves.' Often? I reply, wondering about my fellow humans.

Medea admits that some of her clients are drawn to S&M because they experienced some sort of trauma or abuse as children which they need to keep playing out. But she says many are drawn to it because they feel guilty about wielding so much power.

'One judge who comes here needs to be humiliated. I believe it comes from the exhaustion and responsibility of having to make life and death decisions all the time.

'Many of my clients want to just give up their enormous power and play a different role. They want that relief.' She says that one of the favourite fantasies of powerful, straight men is that the woman straps on a dildo, and acts out a dominant male role with them.

Medea says all mistresses are trained as submissives first so they can understand their clients' deepest needs. 'We go on a psychological journey with our clients.'

Medea claims to have the total support of the surrounding neighbours. 'This used to be a squat house before, with lots of noise. We are quiet and discreet.' Also she says she supports the local establishments like the hardware store where she gets all her leather for the whips and wood for her racks.

One of Medea's mistresses makes dolls for children in her spare time. At least two are also journalists, one of whom I know quite well from her past profession. It's good to know that if one ever gets tired of lashing one's subjects with words, there is always a new, more literal place for old journalists to go to mete out our punishment.

SEX-TOYS

My husband is not at all well. He is curled up on the couch sulking. He claims to be in substantial pain as a result of our last night's activities.

It's all my fault. I was inspired by the latest survey out of America 'Toys In the Sheets'.

According to the survey, which was done for the most recent meeting of the Society for the Scientific Study of Sexuality, the typical owner and buyer of sex-toys such as vibrators is not the young and hip swinger of popular imagination. Rather a sober, married, educated and probably Christian, middle-class white woman, in her thirties – generally with children.

Her household income is between $50,000 and $70,000 and she is most probably a conservative voter. In the USA she votes Republican. Here she would be a Liberal or National Party voter.

Well-regarded San Francisco medical writer Michael Castleman who co-wrote the survey with the Lawrence Research Group says the study, which was conducted on existing sex-toy owners across America, suggests 'that sex-toys are not weird fetishes. They are used by people in the ordinary middle classes, by the family next door.'

Jo-Anne Baker, who runs The Pleasure Spot in Sydney and sells mail order sex-toys all over Australia, agrees. 'My clients are both men and women. Many of them are average family people with children. I get a lot of corporate women buying vibrators and a lot of men coming in to buy them for their wives.

'I would agree that sex-toys are increasingly selling to the mainstream rather than to fringe groups – particularly with sex-shops for women opening up all over the world and pro-viding a softer option than traditional hard-core sex-shops.'

Most people surveyed said they did not use sex-toys as a substitute for sex, with most being married or in de facto rela-tionships and having sex two to three times a week. Sex-toys were largely used in the bedroom but a surprising number of people used them in a host of exotic locations including in cars, tents, spas, a golf course, an aeroplane and surprisingly, a chair lift.

Anyway, the thing that got my husband and I going were the glowing testimonies at the back of the study from sex-toy users.

'Sex-toys saved our marriage!' says one woman. 'We couldn't live without them,' says another. 'The variety keeps married sex-life fun, interesting, exciting and creative…with awesome orgasms.'

It was the awesome orgasms that got me. I insisted we road-test these devices before I wrote this piece. So off we went to get some toys in Sydney's famous Kings Cross.

For those who haven't ventured into a sex-shop, the typical, hard-core store is more like a ghoulish wax museum than a house of erotica. There are too many dismembered body parts behind glass showcases or hanging on the wall, to be a turn-on.

My husband was most upset by the battery-operated *squirming finger* for girls. He was also a bit horrified by the *vibrating tongue* for women which was a bit of pink plastic poking out of a painted mouth with teeth. Meanwhile, I was mortified by the female heads hanging off the walls around the room like a scene from a guillotine horror film.

'We call this male sex-toy the "tunnel of love" the man behind the counter offered, without a sense of humour. 'This is the Trudy model,' he said pointing to a brunette head with an open mouth. 'This is Jennifer,' he said pulling down a pouting blonde and handing it to my husband who gasped as he threw the thing on the counter.

We laughed at the fur-lined handcuffs, edible undies, and genital-shaped food moulds to make penis pasta or chocolate *bosom* biscuits – just the thing for our next dinner party. We also giggled at the range of vibrators, most of which were big enough to excavate a road – a typical male view of what females want.

In the end we selected a vibrating butterfly for me, and a vibrating love tunnel for him, thankfully one without the face.

The evening started well enough. My butterfly was providing quite a bit of enjoyment fluttering about until suddenly it short-circuited. Unfortunately some of the cheaper devices can burn-out on lusty women. So we focused our attention on the tunnel of love.

But we realised – alas, too late – that it was too tight. My poor hubby was literally trapped inside the tunnel of love.

We spent the next hour running around in a terrible panic trying to prise the thing loose, until I remembered an old trick I use when I can't get the lid off the pickled-cucumber jar. I run it under warm water which makes something expand or shrink or whatever.

Thankfully it worked, but not before we'd both done a lot of praying. It is little wonder such a huge percentage of sex-toy users – over 90 per cent of those surveyed – believe in God.

STEALING FOR A FIGHT

Don't be alarmed if you hear the neighbours yelling at each other or you see her tossing his prized record collection into the street. It may look like bad news but chances are your neighbours are just doing the dance of love.

After writing about what strange things got people hot, I was amazed to find the amount of readers who confided to me that good argument was one of the biggest turn-ons to their relationship. Stirring the pot, and all that. Many people claimed to be happy in their relationships because they fought, not despite it.

So are humans born to bicker? Apparently we are – from the time sperm starts chasing the reluctant egg around the womb, according to the sexperts.

The respected Janus Report on sexual behaviour claims that a whopping quarter of all women and a third of all men surveyed declared that the best way to make up after an argument is to have a hot, lovemaking session. This led researchers to conclude '…many couples will provoke a fight to attain the subsequent sex.'

Meanwhile, an American study on file with the Family Planning Association of New South Wales called Shared Intimacies – Women's Sexual Experiences concluded: 'Some women mentioned that their highest sexual experiences occurred after an intense argument or fight. Emotions are [often] aroused to a high pitch.'

Rebecca, thirty-two and married for five years, says: 'I realised that sex is often best for me after an argument or fight. I think it may have something to do with...the energy that comes with emotions like hatred and anger that can be transformed into a powerful sexual experience.'

Victoria-based psychologist Desiree Saddik says: 'For some couples arguing is like a game, marking out territory and boundaries. It is about control and desire, and most of all rage.

'This can be very sexually arousing particularly in certain cultures. All that blood pumping can physiologically resemble a state of lust. And angry women can really turn some men on – the heaving breast, the flared nostrils. There is something exciting in it, something dangerous. It's like the woman is an animal on heat.'

While this is all very good for the male, experts aside, I am not convinced that arguing is necessarily a turn-on for most women.

Despite the flushed cheeks, racing heart and flared nostrils, when I am angry with my partner I think more about thumping him than pumping him.

When voices get raised in our house it is not often the precursor to love. At least not until my husband has apologised for something he either did or didn't do (an irrelevant detail for most women), bought flowers and then, just for good measure, apologised again.

The point of the gift bearing and elaborate apologies is to dissipate the anger which I believe is the single biggest killer of libido in most women.

Angry women can go without sex for weeks, months even years in order to prove to the person that they are really, really, really, pissed off! Far from falling into the arms of a man who has inflamed and impassioned her during a fight, a woman is more likely to push him away and send him off to rectify the offending situation.

He: 'My darling. You look so sexy with your nostrils flared. Let us away to the bedroom!'

She: 'You go back and fix the washing machine the way it says in the manual. I'm sick of washing clothes by hand.' By the time the offending problem is fixed, and many, many apologies have been made, those wild surges of testosterone have vanished into the twilight zone.

Anne Hollonds of Relationships Australia in New South Wales is apt to agree with me. She says although a significant number of the couples do fight habitually to inspire sex and passionate making-up sessions, she believes they are in a destructive relationship and probably frightened to get close.

Meanwhile Queensland sex therapist Dr Diane Meehan agrees anger dampens arousal for many women even though she believes the emotional intensity does probably inflame the ardour of a lot of men. She thinks that for women, sex after arguments is often the result of wanting to get away from the discomfort of the unresolved conflict – a form of procrastination or a yearning for reassurance – more than anything more romantic.

The thing the experts all agree on is that arguing is healthy if done to promote an exchange of views rather than as a form of put-down. Constant bickering and demeaning one's partner, or physical aggression, are the killers of libido not a bit of verbal fisticuffs.

But is it really a turn-on? Saddik says yes. Couples who never fight and who are conflict aversive can become depressed because their relationship never gives rise to heat and desire, and never carries the risks of daring to express a differing view. 'People get bored in a completely perfect, ideal world,' she says.

KINKY KINDS

I once asked a boyfriend what he fantasised about in bed. I wished I hadn't. Without flinching he told me. 'I have a recurrent fantasy. There are cowboys coming over a mountain and they are chasing Indians. Hundreds of Indians wearing big head-dresses,' he said, waving his arms about and puffing his chest like a warrior.

I figured he hadn't heard the question. 'I didn't ask you what you watched on television last night. Do you fantasise about other women?'

'No,' he said, very alarmed that I couldn't see the immediate sexual appeal of the scene he had created.

Years later, after he had galloped on out of my life, I brought this up with my therapist. I asked her if she thought it strange that a person get turned on by such a thing. She said absolutely not. She explained to me that people get turned on by the strangest things often related to their childhood experiences.

If, for instance, someone is experiencing sexual feeling when they are young and they feel guilty about it, they may displace that feeling onto a nearby object. Like an orange juicer. Thereafter always getting aroused by the sound of oranges being squished. Or they may be watching mother doing housework and instead of acknowledging their Oedipal feelings, they may project them onto the vacuum cleaner. Apparently this is quite common.

Many people don't even know what is turning them on in later years. They may suddenly feel aroused eating an ice cream or watching *Mr Ed* on TV.

The conversation with my therapist came to mind recently when I read that prominent psychologist and social commentator Hugh Mackay had, in his novel *Little Lies*, written about a man who could only reach orgasm while holding a train ticket in his hand. So I decided to do a quick ring around of some therapists, sex counsellors and fantasy workers to find out what really turns people on. And the results are quite amazing.

According to the experts, forget the bubble baths, sexy lingerie, chocolates and champagne touted in glossy magazines. It's more likely to be the Hills hoist, or our favourite pink blanket from yesteryear that gets us hot.

Apparently, it's all to do with the safety and security of home or the latent yearnings of childhood. As I wrote last week, according to a recent study by the Smell & Taste Treatment & Research Foundation in Chicago perfumes produced only a 3 to 4 per cent increase in male arousal compared to 40 per cent for the homely blend of doughnut and black licorice, lavender, and pumpkin pie.

Mundane, boring domestic appliances are the subject of many fantasies that Sandra Van Dijk, a former journalist, has to handle each day as Mistress Medea. Van Dijk claims that one of her clients gets turned on watching her put flowers in a vase.

'It's definitely something to do with mother. I think it makes him feel safe. Or maybe he had his first orgasm whilst staring at a vase. Who knows? I'm afraid to ask,' she says.

Another client gets excited by shirts. He likes to hold them close to his body and even glues buttons to the hair on his chest to remind him of shirts, before he can perform.

The funniest of her stories is a man who is fixated with carpet. He carries around a large square of it and often lies under it at parties. Van Dijk says the fellow comes over to her fantasy house each week, and pays $300 an hour to curl up near the front door. He also gets sexually aroused by doormats, and watching women wipe their feet.

If this is all a bit too much, I have just finished reading a fair dinkum psychological report about a man who became sexually excited by his secretary because she waddled. He kept bragging about how beautifully she walked, imitating her and carrying on about the way her feet turned out.

Later it was revealed that he had a sexual fixation with ducks. It was something in the movement of their bottoms.

Melbourne psychologist Desiree Saddik has also heard stories of people who were aroused such exciting and sexy things as toothpaste – 'the association of going to bed.'

She says many men and women are apparently aroused by blankets, thermometers or things to do with doctors and sickness because when they were sick as kids they were given a lot of love and cosseting. 'It is often the intimacy they crave as children and later in life this translates into sexual feelings.'

Other things she has heard of include bad breath. 'Often if a parent has alcohol or cigarette breath, and the child is in an Oedipal phase, this will translate to a life-long arousal trigger,' Saddik says.

I know of two cases of being aroused by cupboards. One girlfriend's husband used to lick cupboards to get himself in the mood. Another woman likes to hide in them before sex.

The strangest story came from Sandra Van Dijk who has a client who gets aroused by excessively hairy arms and pimply bottoms. Which certainly proves that humans are a complex lot when it comes to sexuality. Otherwise put: 'One man's trash is another man's treasure.' Now I'm going off to crawl back under the doormat.

NOISY NEIGHBOURS

Undoubtedly one of the most awful experiences known to man is finding yourself living next door to noisy neighbours.

The sense of powerlessness as the rock music thuds its ugly beat through the night, the knots in the pit of the stomach as bratty children run around yelling and shrieking, the annoyance of having to listen to someone else's TV show as it wafts through open windows or, worse, their mundane domestic fights – these are the sounds that urban nightmares are made of.

But all these horrors pale in comparison to the ultimate aural curse – the neighbour who is noisy in the sack.

There is nothing as infuriating, intimidating or embarrassing as hearing your noisy neighbour sigh and moan in ecstasy for hour after hour while you lie there looking up at the ceiling wondering why on earth you never had sex like that.

Then you think maybe you did have sex like that. But when? And if you did have sex like that, why can't you remember it? Was it ever so good that you moaned and groaned and yelled in passion for so many hours that the neighbours had to put pillows over their ears?

We once lived next door to a woman who made such a fracas it woke us up every morning. She'd let out piercing shrieks that registered ten on the Richter scale. In the beginning we would lie there and giggle softly, amused at the din. Sometimes we'd even feel inspired ourselves. But after the novelty wore off it became downright irritating – a testimony that commented on our sex-life, or rather lack of it at 6am.

'Oh, no! Not again', I'd grumble in my sleep as she'd go off again for the third time in a row like one of those alarm clocks that goes silent for a few minutes but then starts up again in case you've gone back to sleep.

'She couldn't be...' my husband would grizzle pulling the doona over his head and hoping I didn't dive over the fence in search of the stud who could give a woman that much pleasure. Actually she shared with two men which certainly had me thinking.

'She must be faking it,' I'd answer from my sleep. 'She's an actress for sure,' he'd say. But really we were shaken to the core that such pleasure was possible.

Indeed my husband and I both got smitten with 'noise envy' – a potent, destabilising modern affliction, as yet undiagnosed by yuppie shrinks, that drives thousands of people out of perfectly good marriages each year, in search of passionate carnal delights they believe *other people* are having.

But those with noise envy can relax. Having had a discussion with the experts, I have discovered that there is no medical correlation between the amount of pleasure one experiences and the amount of noise one makes.

Psychologists argue it all boils down to personality, how emotionally repressed you are, and how much noise you made in your formative sexual years, whether you feared getting caught.

But international sexpert Barbara Carrellas has a different theory. She says it's all about what sort of orgasm you prefer.

Carrellas who regularly tours Australia from the United States is a teacher of sexuality who specialises in helping people have better orgasms. She says there are many different ways to experience sexual ecstasy.

For instance, if a person remains very quiet before and during orgasm and concentrates on the build-up of sexual energy, he or she is likely to have a very intense 'genital-based' orgasm.

This differs markedly from what is known in the Eastern

lovemaking tradition of Tantra as the *full-body orgasm*. If the person is a screamer, then he or she will most likely be inadvertently hyperventilating – drawing a lot of oxygen into the body with every moan or scream. Oxygen changes the way the muscles respond to pleasure and hence gives a person a very different type of orgasm.

Instead of holding the breath and tensing against the orgasm, the person is letting go. All the muscles in his or her body are relaxing due to the oxygen intake which allows energy to move up the torso like a giant wave and results in a more consuming experience.

Having recently done one of Carrellas' Tantra workshops, it is clear that *full-body orgasms* are surprisingly less draining than the intense genital-based orgasms. In fact, you feel energised and invigorated afterwards, which accounts for why screamers are often at it again ten minutes later. But it's all really just a matter of taste – so to speak.

Carrellas says for those who want to know in advance how noisy their new love will be, they should observe what happens on a dinner date when the food arrives.

Does the conversation suddenly go silent while he or she concentrates on each mouthful, or is there a lot of chatter and breathing between bites? If the latter is the case, you may wish to buy your neighbours some earmuffs in advance.

FAT BOYS

I have always loved fat on men. 'Schmaltz' as it is known in Yiddish and German. 'Voluptuous curves' as the condition was known in Renaissance times. Rubens and I would have been great mates, admiring together the glowing roundness of fleshy thighs, tummies and breasts.

I adore chubby, inviting arms. But I am most partial to fat bellies. Bellies that tell of overindulgence, of overeating. Bellies that tell of long nights spent in hedonistic pursuit with not a thought spared for that enemy of the fat cell – exercise.

I have never had anything but admiration for those orgiastic souls who have – as my mother always disapprovingly described it – 'let themselves go'.

The mere concept of total unrestraint has always whetted my ardour. Men who don't give a brass razoo what society dictates is etiquette and elegance. Men with unrestrained hair, appetites and emotions who cry in sad movies and never, never say no to oily chips, blocks of chocolates consumed in midnight feasts, and plenty of plonk. Men who only jog to catch the Mr Whippy ice cream van before it drives off. To me a bit of schmaltz speaks of abundance, potency, fertility but most of all fun.

But having outlined in almost scientific detail the reason for my penchant, I must pose a question. I know why I like fat men, but what is the excuse of other women I talk to? Because lately I have discovered a most interesting and provocative new trend. Many, many of my women friends are increasingly admitting to me that they too secretly love fat men. Not your obese, ten-tonne monster mind you, rather a voluptuous, curvaceous ball of fleshy manhood. 'Warm and cuddly', was how one girl put it.

In the middle of a radio interview with comedienne Wendy Harmer, she revealed: 'I adore fat men. Men with cute bellies poking out over the pants.' She said every time she went out to lunch she scoured the room for them.

During a recent dinner with a psychologist girlfriend of mine, I heard how much she missed her ex-boyfriend's bulging belly. 'It was so cute,' she sniffed. And to top it all off, two girl-friends admitted to me in separate instances last week that while their romantic fantasies concern slim, traditionally attractive men, their sexual fantasies often focus on fatter, larger men.

This is not the first time I have heard this. Countless books and articles written about women's sexual fantasies have confirmed that many women get turned on by schmaltzy men. Certainly enough women have told me this over the years.

Why? The psychologist I went for dinner with claimed the phenomenon was Oedipal. That many women still yearned for that large, cuddly father figure. To a child, Daddy was always big and bulky because the little girl was so small during her Oedipal phase. Adult women often still carry this image of Daddy with them, and schmaltz can trigger in them feelings of perceived childhood safety.

She said some other women may subliminally be identifying with the concept of abundant, pregnant bellies. A girlfriend reckons it is because a lot of women like to see themselves as smaller than men. So a large man will make them feel petite, frail and feminine.

Meanwhile another leading Australian psychologist, whose clients include some of the country's leading business men and women, says that many women are still subconsciously attracted to the connotations of power carried in the image of a man with an overtly active appetite.

She said that while recent studies of women's sexual fantasies have indicated that today's younger women aspire to dominate men in bed, many baby-boomer women still felt guilty and uncomfortable with their newfound power. During the day they were superwomen, balancing the demands of career, home and children on their shoulders. But at a deep subconscious level they craved a man after dark who would snatch from them the ominous burden of responsibility. Who would take control. Make all the decisions and often forcefully relieve them of a heavy load.

Thus women often sought the psychological as much as physical engulfment that a large, strong or portly male could bring.

Interestingly enough a male friend – who grew up with three sisters – summed it up like this. 'Perhaps the attraction many women have to fat men is that a woman always wants someone who will love her as she is and not be put off by her wrinkles, crinkles, cellulite or pregnant tummy. Imperfect men provide a welcome relief from judgment.'

He says that an interesting point which is often overlooked by the media is that a lot of men do also secretly have attractions to voluptuous women for the same reasons. 'I know men romanticise about the slim, perfect woman, but I believe that a lot of men are also often sexually enchanted by the imperfect because the imperfect enhances their own sense of manhood, security and potency rather than having performance anxiety in the face of a young, spunky, perfect lover.'

He says that many men also yearn to abdicate responsibility and control in bed to a strong, buxom woman which is why so many politicians and leading entrepreneurs keep getting caught in embarrassing S&M type situations. Men also have Oedipal feelings tied in with a large-breasted mother, he claims.

In light of all this it seems very strange to me that we all fast, diet and starve ourselves down to nothing, men and women alike, myself included, in a bid to please the opposite sex. Perhaps fashion will once again dictate a return to Rubenesque roundness. Perhaps aerobics will once and for all be outlawed.

There'll be abundance throughout the land. The catch-cry of the '90s may well end up being: Viva la schmaltz-ball!

SEX FOR ONE

One of the greatest taboos in society still remains the act of self-pleasure. In fact you can't even call it by its proper name. Just mention of the 'M' word and people turn puce and start fidgeting. So I wasn't at all surprised by the reaction I got from friends when I did two workshops which focused on the 'P' words – private parts and pleasure.

One was a workshop on erotic massage: two days of intense investigation into how to turn your partner on. And I'm not talking about wearing sexy lingerie.

The other was the girls-only workshop I described earlier called *Sex-for-One*. Self-loving taken to the extreme! Very voguish in America with post-modern feminists all looking up their own dresses and seeking out their G spots, but still very taboo here. This was the one that most shocked my friends. They glared at me like stunned mullets when I told them what I had spent the weekend doing.

Who in their right mind would spend two days learning how to pleasure oneself? What is there to learn? And anyway, who would feel justified in indulging in two days of intense self-love? Above all, who would do such a bizarre thing in front of a group of strangers? Well, of course, I would. And it was fantastic.

From both workshops I learned secrets about the male and female anatomy that stunned me. Wisdoms that were passed down in ancient cultures from mother to daughter and father to son, but that in Western society continue to elude us.

Sadly, there is no mechanism in our culture to help us see sex as a positive force. No sexual initiation rites that educate us to the powers of our body, and the potential our bodies have for pleasure.

But it was the *Sex-for-One* course that had the most profound effect on me. It allowed me to see how 'pleasure negative' we really are in this society.

It is considered quite normal in this culture to feel bad about touching our bodies, looking at them, enjoying them. We feel sickened at the thought of experiencing too much pleasure or loving ourselves too much. It is as if there is only a certain quota of joy owing to us.

More significantly, in Judaeo-Christian-based societies, we tend to feel that our pleasure has to be reliant on another person. In fact, in the natural order of things, it very often isn't. There are times when we feel intensely sexual but we don't want to be touched by our partners.

There are many reasons for this. The most common being that we see our partners every day. We are intimate on so many levels that we often go into overload. We often just want to retreat into our fantasies much the same way as we turn on the television or read the paper, at the exclusion of our partners.

This *time out* is a normal and healthy occurrence for both men and women, particularly in long, live-in partnerships like marriage. It has nothing to do with love or the lack of it. And it is an enormously liberating experience to be able to distance ourselves for a while, without guilt.

Yet there is a huge stigma in telling our partners that we don't feel like sharing our sexuality with them for a time. There is an equally huge stigma about talking to our friends about it. Luckily for me I have a plethora of very open and honest friends who have joked with me about this rarely discussed penchant many couples have for occasionally going it alone.

What intrigues me is that so many of us still don't trust the wisdom of our own bodies. Too many people are still trying too hard to live by rules that are set down by 'other people' – rules on how we are supposed to experience sex, marriage or pleasure, how our bodies are supposed to look, how we are supposed to touch our bodies or our partner's bodies, and how often.

We're not encouraged to explore our bodies. We are not encouraged to discuss the truth behind many of the myths, and we are certainly not encouraged to listen to our own instincts. Hence, we deny ourselves the things we need when it comes to pleasure, particularly self-pleasure.

What struck me during the Sex-for-One workshop was how much more tolerant we are of pain than joy. Each night on TV we watch people in their death throes. We witness people's most intimate painful moments: suffering, or dying whilst loved ones scream and cry. Yet to watch other people having pleasure is still so forbidden and so taboo.

Through these workshops I have now witnessed people experiencing pleasure – with partners or alone – and it was beautiful and spiritual. I know I'll get a swathe of furious letters from that statement. One woman wrote recently that I should be put into an asylum.

Perhaps she's right. But aren't we all tired of the so-called normality of violence, deprivation, self-hatred, cruelty and pain? Where is the pleasure lobby? Maybe I'll form my own Pleasure Positive Party and I'll force everyone to have a few hours of wanton, abundant, meaningless joy before they come to lock me up and throw away the key.

THE RATING GAME

I was having drinks with some old girlfriends the other night and we did what girls are apt to do when they've had a few too many drinks – we compared notes on the lovers we had shared during our single years.

Over a couple of bottles of chilled white, and with a great deal of laughter, we decided to rate our various 'conquests in common' from one to ten. This of course may come as a nasty shock to men who tend to think that giggling girls in groups are discussing fashion. In fact, women discuss sex far more than the men I know ever do. And we are a far raunchier lot than men are, at that.

Anyway back to our discussion. The interesting thing is that a lover who I rated a four without flinching, actually rated ten with another one of my friends. Then one who I rated ten-plus, was demoted to a mere three by a couple of his former girlfriends.

The very reason I rated him a ten was the reason they rated him a three. I adored the fact that he was into erotic things. It took him ages to get to the actual business of sex. He delighted in hours of delectable teasing and mind games. He loved fantasies and exploration. When he finally got to the act, he wasn't what we girls call a 'stayer' but by that stage I had had such fun, I hardly noticed.

In complete contrast these two were complaining that he took ages to get to the real stuff of sex and then 'conked out'.

This conversation, together with a survey that was released recently by Durex, the condom makers, got me thinking. According to Durex's global survey, the French are considered to be the best lovers in the world whilst the Poles are the worst.

But what really is a 'good lover' if one person's trash is clearly another's treasure? There is a simple answer to this vexing question, according to psychologists. Contemporary New

Age wisdom has people falling into three basic psychological categories: those who are visual, those who are aural–verbal, and those who are sensual.

Being a visual person means you tend to speak in terms of: 'I see what you mean', whereas an aural–verbal person will say: 'I hear what you are saying'. A sensual–feeling person will often say: 'I understand where you are coming from', or 'I relate to that'.

Although most of us have all three characteristics, one is the dominant orientation, with many people also having a very strong second trait. For instance, I am a very aural–verbal type with a strong visual orientation. This is a common makeup for writers.

How does this relate to sex? Quite logically. In the case of the guy I rated number ten and myself, we were clearly into the same sorts of things: fantasies, word games and visual delights. Not surprisingly, he was in the communications industry.

The other two women are predominantly sensuous. They need to feel skin against skin, body against body in order to have any joy in the sex act. They love to be held and touched. They also need to be told 'feeling' things in bed, words that denote tenderness.

Whilst this fellow enjoyed the physical exchange of sex, he was clearly spinning out with pleasure well before it ever even got to the point of touch. The way a woman's body curved, the way she looked in sexy lingerie, the sound of a deep and throaty laugh would be enough to thrill him.

Interesting he also used to ring up phone-sex hotlines. The girls were aghast when they discovered this, describing him to me as 'kinky' and 'bizarre'. I was not alarmed, having always understood why certain people enjoy phone-sex, erotic stories, sexy lingerie and videos, and various other visual and aural accessories to sex.

I use the word 'people' because I think it is a myth that men are basically into emotionally detached sex, whilst women are the feeling ones. Again it depends on which category you fall into.

I have known many men who need to feel connected both physically and emotionally during sex and who shun erotic movies because they have no deep and meaningful plot. And I know plenty of women who get turned on without a shred of emotion. It's just that it is socially unacceptable for women to admit this.

The theories on people's psychological orientations go a long way to explaining the huge gulf between many lovers and why the notion of being universally 'good in bed' is so stupid.

In my opinion the only universal thing that makes someone good in bed is a willingness to accept differences in their partner and not get all insulted if he needs the visual stimulation of sexy lingerie, or get frustrated if she would rather experience sex as an act of love.

A good lover will indulge their partner generously and, most importantly, without judgment.

PEEPING TOM

What really goes on in the homes of suburban Australia? What do people really say to each other and do to each other?

If one is to believe the tele and the magazine articles that ply the newsstands, there are wonderful, exotic and erotic things happening out there to *other people*.

Other people are having the times of their lives. *Other people* are having affairs with exciting celebrities. *Other people* are travelling. *Other people* are doing drugs, doing time, doing just about anything that is bizarre, out of the ordinary or just plain, old riveting. Most annoying of all, *other people* are having kinky sex, one-hour orgasms and have loads of energy to play all night regardless of children, mortgages or unemployment.

Well, finally, I got fed up with reading about *other people* with long legs, straight teeth, and large wallets. I got sick of trying to decipher the urban myths from reality. So I have decided to yield to a bad habit I kicked long ago, in a bid to uncover the truth about the Aussie heartland – spying. For the sake of providing an unbiased, empirical bit of reporting, for the sake of all my readers who deserve a realistic picture of what goes on in this country, I have taken my binoculars from their resting place.

Before I start I must say that everything they tell you on *Hard Copy* and other schlock-TV shows about America is true. Having spied on my neighbours for over a year in Manhattan (perving on the neighbours in high-rise apartment blocks is a national pastime) I am happy to report that behind closed doors in Rambo-land *other people* do exactly what you would imagine them to be doing.

For hours and hours I would sit on my balcony in Manhattan and watch the TV-sized windows and what went on in the frame. On a clear night, specially in smouldering, smutty summer, you can watch people make love or have fights. There are countless channels. My friend actually had a powerful telescope so I could study in great detail the Indian fellow opposite who would strip himself naked and then drink himself into oblivion before doing Karma Sutra type things to his wife. I learnt a lot.

There were two prostitutes across the road. I watched in

horror as one woman's pimp dragged her screaming into the street. I saw crack being traded just under my window because the metho clinic was on the corner of my street and addicts were attracted to the neighbourhood. Many of the crack dealers were women with babies in prams. They used their kids as a foil.

The woman next to me was a sex therapist who used to bonk her man on the kitchen table with the blind up. These tales are all true. I justified my rampant voyeurism to myself by claiming it made me a better writer to watch *other people* at life. Except that I never got any writing done because I remained glued to the lens for hours and hours a day, month in and month out. So I had to give up the distracting habit.

But since I have recently moved into a high-rise apartment in a high-density area of Sydney surrounded by hundreds of windows, and since I now feel it is my duty to ascertain the truth, I prop myself up in a comfortable position, binoculars focused, and prepare for the worst. I expect to see drugs, orgies, wife swapping – all the things they tell you in magazine and tele stories are happening out there in the Aussie suburbs to *other people*.

Things start slowly. The man across the road is out all day. At night he comes in, scratches his privates, eats an apple, opens his mail and plonks himself in front of the television with his cat. This routine occurs most nights of the week. On Saturday night a lady comes over. They eat dinner in the kitchen, drink some wine and retire to the television. At 2am, I am dozing and they are still watching videos.

Two doors down I watch a family eat dinner every night. The daughter sometimes dances in her room. The family usually sits in front of the TV until about 10pm then all the lights go out. Downstairs I watch three women who live together. They never have men over. They don't seem to be gay. In fact, there seems to be no sex in this household whatsoever. Just a lot of cooking and washing dishes.

A man and a woman seem to be doing drugs two doors across. He keeps handing her something. She hands it back. After an hour of squinting and hopping about I realise they are playing chess.

A week later and not much has changed. I think I can see wild sex going on in one of the rooms. It looks exciting and passionate. Arms and legs are flaying about. On closer inspection it turns out to be a pink towel hanging over the bath which is being scrubbed by a cleaning lady.

Week three, there has been no kinky sex, no drugs, no Hitchcock-style murders or suicides yet. I determine to give it time. Australians have never been as greedy or self-destructive as the Yanks. They certainly wash a lot of dishes and watch a lot of TV.

Late one Saturday night I watch two chubby women date two chubby men. They start dancing in front of the window – quite frenetically. Suddenly one of the women falls to the floor. Sex. I am about to see sex. Heavy petting. The real thing. The other three suddenly drop too. I see several sets of legs in the air and then I realise what's happening. They are doing exercises. Leg stretches. A sort of dusk-to-dawn aerobics session.

Week four and still nothing for Madonna to put into her next book. Where is the stuff from tele? Where are all the cross dressers and transvestites? Where are those 'other people' who take amphetamines and have threesomes? Are things happening in other rooms of the house: the ones with curtains over the windows, or aren't they happening in the Australian suburbs?

In desperation I sink really low, to eavesdropping. At night I press my glass to the wall next door. She says: 'Do you think the chicken was dry?' He says: 'It was okay.' He says: 'Did you send in the car insurance payment?' She says: 'Yeah.' This is not at the kitchen table but in the bedroom.

Revelation TV has got it all wrong. This is real life. This is the true stuff our lives are made of in Australia. Routine. I'm throwing in my binoculars. I'm going back to the tube. It's far more exciting and unpredictable.

SAFE SEX

We are standing in the kitchen, my husband and I, doing kinky things with last night's dinner. We've taken the leftovers out of the refrigerator and are slowly, sensuously, kissing the plastic wrap covering each of our dishes. He is getting heavy with the chicken, I'm getting erotic with the egg salad.

We are trying hard not to laugh, because this is no laughing matter. I'm doing my research for a story on safe sex and what people are really using out there to protect themselves from disease. The fact is, condoms only serve to protect certain parts of the human anatomy. There are plenty of other places unwanted germs and viruses can enter, particularly the mouth which is very susceptible to cuts, burns or bleeding gums. So, according to a friend who knows, people are experimenting with none other than the trusty kitchen-wrap.

We decide to check it out. But my husband is a passionate man, and suddenly his tongue pierces the kitchen-wrap and plunges head-long into the roast chicken. If the chook had been a genital, he'd be in a lot of trouble.

'That's the problem with kitchen-wrap,' my friend informs me. 'It is sheer which is good for mobility and sensation, but it does tear easily. Try this dental dam,' he says providing us with what looks like a rubber handkerchief.

We take the dental dam home and open the packet. It smells like vanilla which apparently is part of its appeal. It comes with lubricant so that it can be stuck in place. I playfully cover my mouth. My husband, in one gallant movement, sweeps me up in his arms and passionately kisses me on the dental dam.

'Yuk. Oh, yuk,' he whines. 'It tastes like I'm licking a vanilla-flavoured car tyre.' Truth is, it doesn't taste too good from my end either. But I keep thinking about all those horrible viruses that are making their way around the world like sequels to a bad Hollywood movie. You've been scared out of your wits by Hepatitis A, B and C. Now there's D and the brand new Ebola virus coming soon to a body near you.

My doctor tells me that some strains of hepatitis, as well as herpes, gonorrhoea and syphilis, can be spread through saliva. Meanwhile HIV can be caught through oral sex.

STDs are becoming increasingly resistant to antibiotics and penicillin. The question on everyone's lips is: Would you rather have an amoeba eat your brain or perform cunnilingus on a plastic bag? Otherwise put, is sex worth dying for?

'No, No. No,' I yell, pushing the dam off my face, unsure which of the two options I'm protesting most about.

I am saddened to discover how awful these things taste because I have always been a vigilant promoter of safe-sex prac-tices. I have written about them and preached them from the rooftops, albeit from the smugness of a good marriage.

No use telling me that people shouldn't be promiscuous. They are – straight and gay – with statistics suggesting that 40 per cent of Australians have had extramarital affairs at one time or another.

No use telling me teenagers shouldn't have condom machines in schools. Teenagers are amongst the fastest-growing heterosexual HIV carriers in the USA and continue to be a worry in Australia, according to Dr Julian Gold, Director of the Albion Street AIDS Centre in Sydney. Kids do have sex. I have no time for puffy sentimentality or lofty morality in the face of a world-wide plague.

But does safe sex have to feel so bad? One safe sex introduction kit put out by AIDS awareness groups includes a pair of rubber gloves to protect nail biters, and those who are creative with their hands. Whilst playing doctors seems kinky enough, the feel of rubber gloves on one's skin is less than satisfying.

My husband hates condoms, describing them as 'wearing a raincoat two sizes too tight into a bathtub'. Instead he has a safe-sex alternative for me – a female condom brought back from the USA. It's so huge, you could put the scraps from last night's dinner in there and still have room to throw out a few old jumpers you didn't need, and possibly even the weekend papers. It feels as bad as it looks.

Glaring at the chewed up bits of rubber and plastic round the floor, signs of a Brave New World, I am full of dismay.

We do have to practise safe sex. No-one is safe, not even in the sanctity of marriage. AIDS is not just a 'gay' disease and there are plenty of other dangers lurking behind every sexual dalliance.

But personally I'd rather be sentenced to twenty-five years of chastity, and just fantasise about how it used to be in the good old days – hot, juicy sex that did not spell a death sentence, and those wonderful arguments about who slept in the wet spot. Then again, I always was an ol' fashioned gal.

SEX AS A SPECTATOR SPORT

'An increase in decadent behaviour and exhibitionism, boredom with things natural, an obsession with artifice, shocking statements and images, sexual excess.' These are some of the characteristics used by modern dictionaries and encyclopedias to describe the phenomenon known as '*fin de siècle*'.

A French term meaning end of the century, *fin de siècle* came to explain the burgeoning of decadence around the world that erupted as the last century drew to a close.

I find myself thinking more and more about the *fin de siècle* as I venture out into the nightclubs of Australia. It is hard not to wonder, as this turn of the century – indeed the millennium – draws nigh, whether we are not turning into a deeply decadent society.

I visit the hottest 'hot spots' in Australia: the Hellfire clubs. One in Melbourne, one in Sydney. They are doing for S&M in Australia what the Marquis de Sade did for the bizarre practice in Europe. Sadomasochism is being taken out of the closet and on to the streets of middle-class suburbia. Torture, torment and ecstasy for the masses.

Whilst techno-funk music thuds its synchronised industrial sound around a huge warehouse, hundreds of people mill around watching two young girls in school uniform tongue-kiss. A woman in black leather with an executioner's hood over her head drips hot wax down their naked thighs and bums. After the performance, one tells me she is a saleswoman from Tasmania, another is a nurse from Sydney.

I stand with a crowd of seemingly middle-class people watching a woman in leather hitting another woman's breasts with a paddle. I watch a male dominatrix – an interior decorator called Peter – bite another man's naked bum until there are

245

welts everywhere, while the surrounding crowd touch each other, go off into corners and fondle. Go into the bathroom and copulate. Thinly-clad bodies writhe and moan and it is *Caligula* all over again.

In a distant corner, a woman dressed in only kitchen-wrap, leads another near-naked woman on a leash into a corner. They both crouch down and I see nothing but flaying arms and legs between everyone else's feet. I am trembling with shock, with arousal, with confusion. No-one ever told me I'd one day be stepping out of my middle-class home into a porn flick.

A man standing next to me says that he is the father of a four-year-old girl. He's a professional man of forty-two. A regular, he has been coming to the club to watch for months. He says it turns him on. But after talking to him for twenty minutes it becomes clear to me that the recent breakdown of his marriage has more to do with it. He seems to be so angry and in so much emotional pain that this scene is probably cathartic.

All week the visions, both erotic and horrific, play on my mind. Why is it happening? What is really happening? Melbourne-based psychologist and student of the *fin de siècle*, Desiree Saddik agrees that as we hurtle towards the end not just of this century but the end of the millennium, we are plunging into another more extreme period of decadence.

Saddik, who works for the Victoria-based Canterbury Family Centre, says: 'At the end of each century a certain madness pervades the human spirit due to feelings of fear that the world we know will disappear. People are full of uncertainty about the future. Identity becomes blurred. There is often death anxiety leading to a fascination with things violent or sexual.

'We can already see the signs of *fin de siècle* reflected in the sudden proliferation of S&M and body piercing into the mainstream, the trend to androgyny and gender bending, the increase in sexual exploration. There's a voyeuristic fascination in erotica, fantasy and flesh – just like at the turn of this century,' says Saddik, whose passion is psychoanalytic thought.

Saddik's words swirl around in my head as I attend a fashion parade that is more about flesh than clothing. Indeed the attire seems to belong more to the darkest dungeons of S&M subculture than to the shopping malls of middle-Australia. And yet hundreds of people have gathered at another of Sydney's nightspots, Sky, to witness a display of the latest fetish clothing hitting retail outlets around the country.

At the stroke of midnight, a tall woman with long, ebony hair and ghoulish, white skin, emerges from a billowing cloud of crimson smoke. She is wrapped in a black PVC corset, metal bra, transparent shorts and impossibly high, black PVC boots. As she minces down the catwalk with a dog collar around her neck to the thud of techno-funk, images of body piercing and tribal scarification flash on to the walls around the room. The crowd screams in delight.

Another cadaver-like woman is ushered out on a leash by a man in a devil-horn helmet whilst another slaps a whip against the behind of a slave. Images reminiscent of Nazi sadism and devil worship are pumped out to an audience seemingly indifferent to the more sinister undertones of their fashion statements.

'We're selling this stuff to the mainstream,' says a cheerful Katy Milroy from The House of Fetish which recently opened up in Sydney to cope with the rising demand for studded dog collars, leather corsets and steel underwear. 'We thought it would mainly be the gay scene and S&M enthusiasts who would be into this but it's everybody. People are walking in off the street. It's so busy, I'm run off my feet.'

She's right about the sudden interest in such attire. So popular has fetish-wear become that Greenpeace has started protesting publicly about the dangers to the environment and body of wearing the artificial PVC. Even conservative department stores are stocking fetish-wear. Former editor of *Mode Australia*, Maggie Alderson, agrees with the *fin de siècle* theory: 'I do believe we are an increasingly decadent culture. It isn't just fetishism but a total exhibitionism that we are witnessing,' she says referring to strip-tease fashion and the proliferation of lap-dancing clubs.

'There is an increase in sexual depravity, perversions and primitive practices like labia piercing. We have run out of other periods to plunder. There are no great challenges for us any more. We have done everything. And what we haven't done we can watch other people doing on TV.

'We are ailing, waning. I feel like we are watching the last of ancient Rome,' she says alluding to the new obsession with the TV program *Gladiators* where sweaty, near-naked men and women compete in a studio arena to the screams of wild crowds. '*Gladiators* is ritual violence. Just like fetishism recalls images of pre-war Germany, *Gladiators* is another icon of a declining culture,' she says.

Having toured the club-scene here and in New York, having consumed copious amounts of literary and visual erotica and interviewed hundreds of people both here and abroad, I have developed a view of my own as to why there has been such a stark increase in things erotic.

Whilst I give much credence to the *fin de siècle* theory, I think that we are witnessing more than that. I think what we are also seeing is the growth of sex as a spectator sport. Not so much a proliferation of true S&M or ritual violence and decadence, rather a look-don't-touch attitude to sexuality in the wake of HIV and the increasing nasties like Hepatitis A, B, C ad infinitum, super-bugs, and serial killers.

Hollywood, with such gems as *Fatal Attraction*, has warned us off casual sex. We are petrified of health risks. The mind has bravely thrown itself in front of our wild, natural instincts in order to protect us from modern dangers to our species.

And the result is the steady burgeoning of burlesque and sex-clubs where people can go to 'watch' safely from the bleachers – spectators to the raunchy, rugged sport of sex. S&M, and fetishism have always excited and titillated. Even those who are not enamoured with the actual practice cannot fail to be aroused witnessing the fondling of naked flesh, and the sexuality of submission.

Movies, both arthouse and mainstream, are growing steamier and seamier. Appetites are whetted for erotic books and stories. Fantasy is back in fashion with the sharp increase in lap-dancing and strip-clubs, and well-known actresses amongst those endorsing the new trend to take it all off. Meanwhile phone-sex lines and videos for men and women are keeping our imaginations tantalised.

We are turning into a culture of voyeurs and exhibitionists. Perhaps the films, music, literature, fashion and other cultural indicators that are feeding us a decadent and erotic image are indeed hailing in the *fin de siècle*. Or perhaps we just feel better playing the part of audience in the increasingly dark, provocative pantomime that sexuality has become.

NAKED IN NEW YORK

'Seesaw's' is a sex-club inside a large warehouse in the lower part of Manhattan. I had rung up an old friend, Andrew, when

I got to New York to see if he minded taking me inside. I told him I was researching for a book. I told him I believed sex had become a spectator sport. Andrew, a former Fleet Street journalist and a typical English cad, who makes a point of hanging out where most decent folk wouldn't be seen dead – agreed.

He said he'd take me clubbing but it would cost me my modesty. To get into some of the more famous clubs, one had to walk around in a state of undress. 'You can keep a towel over you, but people will feel inhibited about making love in front of someone who is fully dressed,' he informed me, still chortling at my claim that I was doing this for 'research' purposes.

I agreed to disrobe and we bowled up at 'Seesaw's' (not the club's real name) at around 11pm. People were queuing up outside a huge double door which had a two-way mirror at the front. Andrew explained the rules: Couples had to come together. No singles were let in. The reason was that the emphasis was on safe sex; BYO partner and condoms.

The thrill was having sex in public, being watched or watching. If couples wanted to engage in some swapping, that was fine. But this was not the free-for-all environment of Plato's Retreat and other infamous sex-clubs like it that thrived during the excesses of the late '70s and '80s. The threat of HIV had closed those clubs down. Promiscuity was out.

'All the new erotic clubs that are opening up around the world are more or less exhibitionist and voyeuristic,' he explained. 'There is a new sexual revolution erupting but the eroticism is in fantasy, masturbation, self-pleasure or self-pain – anything that is sexy but not overly promiscuous,' Andrew said.

He paid the man behind the counter: a hefty $US200 a couple. Safe, horny sex was obviously a sport of the middle-to-upper classes.

Andrew took me straight to the change-rooms so we could take off our clothes. He told me I could wrap a small towel around myself if it made me more comfortable. I undressed, trying to pretend I was going into a sauna. Then stepped out of the change-room with the towel around my midriff. I was used to being topless on Australian beaches but I didn't want to let go of the towel. Or the high-heels. I don't go anywhere I can't wear high-heels.

'Great,' said Andrew who was also in a towel. 'Now we go into the disco area just to peruse the other couples.' He pulled out a bottle of wine he had smuggled in.

The disco area was just like something out of the '70s. A large ball with glass mirrors twirled about in the middle of the ceiling, throwing fragmented light around the room. Some couples were in towels, others totally naked, but some were dressed up to kill. I was immediately horrified by the number of clothed individuals.

'You told me everyone was naked,' I said, growing alarmed. He laughed and poured some wine. 'Come sit on the couch,' he said, leading me to an area facing the dance floor. 'It's cool. Some people like to check each other out in clothes first. All that seduction stuff. Then they take off their things later. You have to be naked to enter the back of the club which has the spa and sex areas. In here it's optional.

'Because we aren't moving on anyone, I didn't think we needed to be dressed. Besides, I thought you'd enjoy the feel of being in a disco naked. Relax. No-one here knows you.'

That was true. I have always believed that our inhibitions about nudity come from being 'seen' or 'recognised' looking other than our perfect best. Women in particular didn't want their large buttocks or thighs to be revealed if they could be hidden under the illusion of an elegant skirt or dress. But when you realised that no-one knew you or would remember a thing you did, inhibitions mysteriously vanished.

The mating rituals around the room were intriguing to watch. The room was filled with Mr and Mrs Suburbia. One woman had on a large, pink, taffeta dress which she probably had from her prom days. Her hair was coiffed 1960s-style. Her husband looked like someone out of an American kids' show: Dennis the Menace's dad, or Mr Brady from *The Brady Bunch*. He had Brylcream through his hair and wore a checked jacket and tie.

Another couple looked a bit more modern but were still 'the people next door'. She was blonde, about forty-five, with lots of diamond jewellery on and a bad facelift. He was podgy and had the hungry look of a salesman. 'These people come in from the boroughs,' said Andrew. 'The B&T people: Bridge and Tunnel people. They come into Manhattan from Brooklyn or Queens. They are suburbanites who are bored after ten or twenty years of marriage, looking for some kicks. Mainly professional.'

While the Bee Gees sang: 'Night fever...night fever...' Mr Brylcream was smiling at Mrs Diamond-necklace and Mr Salesman was trying to crack on to the prom-queen by licking his lips provocatively in her direction. It was hilarious to watch. But then a whole new crowd arrived. A younger, trendier set. The women were drop-dead gorgeous.

'What's this?' I asked.

'The corporate crowd. The women are often callgirls or mistresses.'

There was a dark woman who looked like she had just stepped out of a Hollywood movie – tall, tight mini-skirt, long hair, sultry face. She was with a Latin man who had on the flashy shirt and the big gold chain. 'She's probably his mistress,' said Andrew informatively. 'Puerto Ricans. He probably doesn't swap her. He just likes other men to see him turn her on.'

After an hour of watching the crowd, I was drunk enough to venture back to 'the other part' of the club. People were in the spa although I figured that it couldn't be too healthy to sit in that water.

There was a large room that Andrew dubbed *the orgy room* beside the wet area. It had a sign on the door saying: WEAR CONDOMS. NO ANAL SEX PERMITTED. 'Wonder how they would police that?' I joked.

Everyone was naked although most of the women were still wearing high-heels, even in the swimming pool area. Still playing the mating game as prescribed in women's magazines. The Puerto Rican woman emerged from the change room naked except for her black, suede heels. 'Mama!' said Andrew.

The woman's silky, brown skin looked as if it would feel like velvet to touch. She was perfect. Hypnotically so. Every eye was upon her. She and the man Andrew dubbed 'Carlos' got into the spa. Suddenly twenty other people crammed into the spa. 'See, he loves that. Loves that other people love his lady. It makes him feel so machismo to see other men drool.'

In the *orgy room* couples were beginning to lie down on mattresses which were laid out in a big circle. I was looking forward to being a fly on the wall. To watching sex happening between people. To seeing first-hand what other people really did, and how they did it.

Soon it started. A couple started fondling each other, then another, then another. Doing what they did in the privacy of their bedrooms, publicly. Before long all the beds were moving.

On the roof was a large mirror. I looked up to what looked like the film set of the movie *Caligula*.

On my right was a middle-aged fellow and his wife. The fellow leaned over and placed his hand on my stomach. Andrew leaned across. 'We're just watching,' he said.

'Sure,' said the guy, and went back to fondling his wife. When Andrew got up to go to the toilet, the fellow tried again.

'No, I'm just here to watch,' I said, trying not to laugh at the stupid line. 'Oh!' said the man exclaiming loudly. 'You're Australian.'

He was brimming with excitement. He was truly more excited than anyone else in the room. 'Oh! I love Australia. I've seen *Crocodile Dundee* I and II. I'd love to go there. Maureen, she lives in Australia.'

Maureen looked as excited as her husband. 'I'm Dan,' he said holding out his hand which had been God-knows-where. He didn't notice that I wouldn't shake it as he exuberantly continued: 'And this is my wife, Maureen. I'm a lawyer and Maureen is, well, you know, a housewife. We have two kids. We live in Brooklyn.' He was whispering loudly. I was terrified it would interrupt the orgy. I was more terrified the whole orgy would sit up and start saying things like 'G'day mate' or 'I love Koalas'.

But before he was able to give me a profile of his entire life which was destined to include how many times he saw his therapist, what he did to cure himself of dandruff and how he felt about his mother, Andrew came back and spirited me off to another part of the room.

'Can't let them start talking, bloody Yanks. Once they start they never shut up,' he whispered. 'The one thing Americans love more than food and sex is a good talk.'

I was trying not to laugh. I really wanted to watch. We went up to a balcony where we could watch the orgy from a safe environment.

It was fascinating. But it was more than fascinating. Rather than feeling horrified or turned on by what I was witnessing, I felt oddly moved. People were so free. People were so comfortable with their bodies, not caring if bums wobbled or thighs wobbled or bellies hung down too low. Not caring if dicks weren't big enough or boobs were drooping. Just pleasuring themselves and others in a wonderful love-a-thon. I felt sad that sexual pleasure was still more socially frowned upon than the ugly diet of violence and cruelty we are fed each night on the TV.

I wished I had a video recorder so I could film just the faces and put the images on television all over the world. 'Look,' I would say, 'Witness happiness. Witness joy.' Andrew was amused by my reaction. I must have been the only woman who had gotten emotional in a sex-club. 'C'mon,' he said pulling me up. 'Time to have another drink.'

He took me upstairs to *The Love Fest*. This was an area where people roamed around and just fondled and touched each other, spontaneously, against walls, on the love-seat, on couches.

The blonde with the diamonds came up to me. 'Hi, honey. That's my husband over there. George.' George waved. 'We saw you in the disco. George is a dentist. We're from Connecticut. Anyway, George was wondering if you'd like to join us... if your partner... ummm... doesn't object that is.'

'We're just watching,' said Andrew, politely. 'Oh *hey*. Look, George won't go with her. George just goes with me, but I'd like to go with her, if that's okay,' she said chewing on something which smelt like an orange lolly.

'Sorry, I'm eating candy. I have this awful sore throat. Oh...
Nothing contagious. You know. I mean, you won't get it...just a
cold. Actually I'm almost better,' she said with a twangy drawl. 'I
mean, you know...you won't catch it or anything.'

I was intrigued. Andrew was right. Americans loved to talk.
And I wanted to hear. 'Do you guys come here often?'

'Oh, about once a week. George likes to watch me go with
people...you know...women. He gets bored at home. We
have two kids. They're both at college...Simon is studying law
...ummm...so, you know...George likes somewhere to go
once a week...you know.'

'Do you like it?'

'Well, yeah. Kind of. But, it turns him on so...you know..
.I'm actually very tired tonight. I had a lump on my breast. The
doctor thought it was cancer. It was just a cyst. Thank God. But
he thinks I'm menopausal...I mean my doctor does, not
George. Which...you know...is a bit depressing. I feel quite
low at the moment...' she said, chatting on and on without air
while George waved hopefully. Finally George came over and
introduced himself. I introduced myself and Andrew.

'Oh,' said George in the same gushy twang his wife had.
'You've got a cute accent. Where are you from?'

'Andrew is English. I live in Australia.'

'Oh. I'd love to go to Australia,' he began like the other fellow, talking of his great love for koalas ('they are so cute') and
kangaroos.

'Sorry we have to go now,' said Andrew dragging me away
once again. By this stage I was giggling uncontrollably.

I had had a bit to drink and somehow managed to lose
Andrew by stepping sidewards. So off I stumbled downstairs.
But on the way down I banged head-long into Miss Puerto

Rico. Still in her high-heels. She was leaning against a wall, looking sexy.

'Sorry,' said I, feeling a bit startled. 'That's okay, babe,' she said, running her hands down my hair. 'Why you in such a rush? Stay and talk a while.'

Carlos was standing nearby smoking heavily. He smiled at me and nodded his approval. I felt a twinge of danger but it soon passed. It was like being in shark-infested waters when there was an abundant school of fish around. I presumed I wouldn't be eaten for dinner. I was wrong.

Suddenly I heard Carlos' deep voice. 'Cummon, babe. I wanna love you,' he said, roughly pushing away his woman to get to me.

For a moment I was in shock. Carlos didn't look like the sort of man who took no for an answer. Andrew, who had been watching gleefully from the sidelines, entered the fray. 'Sorry, she's with me,' he said, wrenching me away.

My head was spinning. My eyes were big as saucers. Andrew grinned and dragged me back to the change-room to get dressed.

An hour later we bowled up to another club. This was once a notorious gay haunt. Now it is mixed. We asked the door man to let us peep in just for a comparison.

Cubicles lined the walls, like toilet blocks but with beds in them. A porn flick was playing in one part of the room. The floor was totally transparent and below was a swimming pool. There were ropes hanging off the glass floor. I stood mesmerised looking down at the contorted human shapes as they swung off the ropes and did gymnastic-type sexual things.

I could see people's brains from their posteriors. Just then I caught a glimpse of a man dangling from the rope with several long feathers sticking out of his behind. It was too much to handle. 'Take me home,' I said feeling fatigued, and somewhat battered.

'Tomorrow I'll take you to some really hard-core places,' Andrew said, grinning at me. But as we got in the taxi I just knew that I'd walked as far as I was prepared to walk on the wild side.

DRESSED TO KILL

I once had a girlfriend who would always wear the sexiest lingerie underneath her day-to-day clothing. As well as frilly bras and lacy undies she wore a silk garter belt, suspenders and those old-fashioned pull-up stockings from the '50s with seams up the back of her legs. Everything was of the highest quality, bought in Paris.

She dressed the way men dream we dress in their fantasies, or when they undress us in their minds.

Which makes me smile when I think how men would react to what women really wear under their clothing – the old bra with the torn strap ('Oh, this will do') shrunken knickers ('My goodness! Have we run out of clean clothes this week already?') and the pantyhose with holes and ladders ('Who's gonna see?'). All the mis-matched bits n' pieces thrown together as we dart about the house, shoving food at children, then dashing out the door to the office, to meetings or out to do the shopping.

We only dress in sexy lingerie on hot dates in the hope of getting lucky which deludes the poor dears into thinking that they are going to see us lay down in silk forever more, only to realise in horror that on cold winter nights when the initial thrill of hot love can no longer warm our stony feet and tired legs, that we prefer the comforting feeling of flannelette against our skin. Those wonderful pink and yellow nighties that my long-suffering husband refers to as 'the best form of human contraception ever invented'.

Anyway here was my friend dressed to kill, but the odd thing was that no-one at the time got to see her lingerie. She was going through what we girls call a dry patch – recently separated from her husband, no male company in sight. I only found out about her underwear because we changed at her place before going to a movie. I was astounded that anyone not having an affair would bother to go to that much trouble.

'Why do you wear this stuff?' I asked. 'It makes me feel good,' she said and then went on to explain that if she felt sexy, she was more confident and powerful.

Now, a decade later, a spate of recent surveys in the USA have made it official. I should have ditched my therapist and invested in some French knickers and crimson lipstick. According to these statistics when women feel sexier they achieve more from the bedroom to the boardroom. And they feel sexier when they diet, make themselves up, wear sexy lingerie and exercise, according to one of the researchers involved, Dr Debbie Then.

Dr Then, a psychology PhD from Stanford University who was in Australia last week discussing sex and appearance, is currently finalising a survey on how body image effects women's sexuality. She says that preliminary results have revealed that over 75 per cent of the women she surveyed – married and single – had a sudden hike in sexual activity and pleasure when they changed their hair colour.

'When the women created a sexier image for themselves they felt better and consequently made more of an effort which affected their attitude to sex and the way they performed sexually.'

She says that another recent survey she has analysed showed that women actually had stronger orgasms when they lost weight and started exercising.

'The reason for this was two fold. One was that they were releasing more feel–good chemicals into their bodies. The other was psychological. The women reported that as they lost weight and got fitter, their self-esteem improved and they became more sexually experimental, trying new positions, dressing up in sexy underwear, flirting, showing off their bodies and playing with sex-toys – which increased their enjoyment significantly.'

She said that most interesting was the conclusion that when women felt better with themselves physically they achieved more in all areas of their lives, from the bedroom to the boardroom.

Whilst I have spluttered and laughed my way through a lot of this research I am hard pressed to argue with the results. I can't honestly remember the last time I went into the office or to a party with greasy hair or in a tracksuit. It's just on the home front that I tend to be a little lazy.

But there is an irony in all of this that stops me feeling too bad. Research shows that a vast improvement in looks or body weight will send husbands and boyfriends into a frenzy of inse-curity. Apparently men fear their new, sexier woman will run off.

So I feel justified curling up in bed in my flannelette nightie after a day of stilettos and frilly knickers. Well girls, we can't have our poor partners feeling too threatened, can we?

AROMAS OF LOVE

It seems that one of my letter writers has created quite a stink: literally. A few weeks ago a Ms L. of Mackay in Queensland wrote to me:

'I have a mate who refuses flatly to bathe himself at the end of the day's work. Instead, he goes to bed grubby (even when the fresh sheets are put on the bed) and showers in the morning before work. On top of all this, he expects me to have sex with an unclean body! It is a complete turn-off. Is this the typical Australian male behaviour? What do other readers think about the stink?'

There then followed a barrage of mail, the likes I haven't seen for ages. Women were furiously responding to this very smelly kettle of fish.

Marilyn of Adelaide complained that this wasn't just Aussie behaviour as her English husband refused to bathe after twelve hour shifts because it would wake him up. 'There are no quickies in our house,' she huffed. Meanwhile M. M. from the Sunshine Coast accused Ms L.'s husband of being beastly. 'I feel sorry for her. She needs to put her foot down or their relationship is doomed. How can he be so selfish to expect her to be turned on by him like that?'

Anon. of Toowoomba theorised that Ms L.'s husband secretly had a low libido and was trying to drive her away with his pong. But a very angry Amy of Keysborough in Victoria lamented the lot of women:

'We poor females are expected to tease and tantalise with the latest fashions, so is it too much to ask our men to go to bed with at least a clean body and clean face? Dirt, sweat and sex just doesn't mix. So all you guys out there who expect the best of us, "clean up your act".'

I have been very much enjoying the response and would like to add my voice to the growing throng about pong. Men have always made women feel very self-conscious about our own smells. The amount of ghastly, sickly-sweet perfumes and feminine hygiene products on the market are a testimony to how neurotic females have been made to feel about their natural odours.

I once went out with a man who, before the lovemaking act, handed me a bottle of green liquid. 'To put you-know-where,' he said looking at my privates. 'It makes women smell beautiful like plants.'

I threw the bottle back in his face and walked to the door. 'If women were supposed to smell like plants, then God would have made us that way,' I said storming into the street, never to see him again.

My female readers are forever complaining that it is very annoying to be expected to smell beautiful, keep your figure, always look magnificent and yet be confronted time and again with men who don't seem to give a hoot about how they look or how they smell.

I am not suggesting that men smell bad. Heavens, no. There are many women out there who go bananas over male smells and find them frighteningly erotic. But I think it is a matter of degrees on the smell-o-meter.

For instance, there is nothing in the world that gets me more excited than the pungent scent of male armpits. But what I am after is a 'force five' on the smell-o-meter – that means somewhere in the middle.

A freshly washed male armpit probably rates a 'force two'. By mid-morning on a hot day, it is getting up around the four mark. By lunchtime, presuming the fellow came into work in an air-conditioned car, not on the train which would accelerate the sweating process, it would just be hitting the five mark. Bingo.

Six is still tolerable but not pleasant. Anything getting close to seven is getting into migraine territory for me. By nine or ten, I am likely to faint on sight.

My husband has learned to monitor his own armpit. He will walk in from work and announce 'force nine' and head straight for the shower. Or he will grin and approach me with his pit in the air, knowing full well that I am about to be over-come with passion and lust.

Whilst I have a high tolerance of armpit, I personally can-not tolerate even a 'force one' in the smelly feet department, and feel ill at even a hint of onion breath.

But even with these most woofie pongs, I am not saying that all men have to be squeaky clean. Perish the thought. The only thing worse than onion breath is the saccharine smell of perfume or aftershave on a man's skin.

It is going to the other extreme to be overly hygienic and to wash away all those fabulous pheromones. Americans, for instance, recently cited bathing as their favourite form of fore-play in a survey, whilst most English people polled said that after sex the first thing they did was run to the bathroom to scrub up. Which brings to mind the word 'sterile'.

Many women I know adore the natural, earthy scent of men, and cannot get passionate with men who smell too sweet.

The point is that where smell is concerned every woman has her own tolerance level and should be respected for that. I doubt a man would let a woman get away with smelling any-thing less than what he could tolerate. We've always prepared ourselves for delicate male nostrils. It is what men have come to expect of us.

Now we're telling you what we expect of you. By all means work up a sweat. By all means produce those male smells that we love at our deepest, primordial levels. But remember to check our Richter scales every now and again.

SLAVE TO LOVE

American television is superbly audacious. One of the funniest, most outrageous programs I have ever watched was a recent talk-back show (screened here late at night) discussing how often couples should or do make love.

I sat boggle-eyed as people stood in front of millions and millions of viewers, all over the world, and discussed their most intimate, private sexual secrets.

The first couple got up to share their nuptial experience. The man volunteered: 'She only wanted it three times a week. I needed it about seven, or more.'

She: 'Yes, but I was tired. I had to stay home with two babies all day. Try feeling sexy after that!'

He: 'Anyway we compromised. Now we do it four times a week – sometimes five.' Pan to the audience, obviously touched by the sincerity of the admission. People start clapping, roaring and cheering in support.

'Thankyou. Thankyou for sharing,' said the TV host, herself clapping to the guests.

Next came a woman who decided to share her secret with the world. She wasn't getting enough.

'Is your husband okay about you coming on the program?' the host asked the scantily clad lady.

'No. I think he's a bit upset,' said the woman to a billion people. She then went on to describe the various techniques she used each night to get her husband in to bed.

'I often stand in sexy underwear while I fry his dinner. Or run around in little outfits with stockings and things...you know. It's never helped much.'

'How often does he make love to you?' asked the interviewer without flinching.

'About five times a year,' came the reply. There was a huge rumble from the audience as the camera made its way up the aisles to show all the shaking, disapproving heads. Bad, bad Mr John Brown from Illinois who now has to seek counselling – not only for his sexual problem but on how to show his red face in public.

Jokes aside, frequency of sexual activity is fast becoming an obsession in the States. In fact it is over-running other sexually related issues such as date rape, sexual harassment at work, and celibacy as the national preoccupation.

Americans are incurable curious people and it is just no longer feasible for them to walk around the streets not knowing what really happens in the beds of their neighbours, their friends and their relatives.

They want to know, once and for all, if they are missing out on something, and if they should be feeling cheated or inadequate.

The trend has also focused attention on the hottest new neuroses. The term being bandied around is 'sex addict', which is used to describe people who have too much sex.

Articles by well-known psychologists and social observers have begun appearing in magazines and newspapers condemning excessive sexual activity. And in keeping with the mania that surrounds any new American trend, scores of people each week are appearing on the tele confessing to extreme and often vulgar behaviour. 'I am a love-a-holic which means I need to have sex ten times a day.' It is intriguing viewing but it has upset many people who now fear themselves to be sex addicts.

The question on everyone's lips is: Am I doing it too much? Am I in love or am I a perverted addict who needs to shoot up on sex? How often is too often? How many is too many? Am I a bonk-a-holic escapist? Do I need help?

And there is help on the way, at a price. Apparently, clinics have started opening up to deal with a problem which has been deemed psychological rather than physical. The clinics are a kind of sexual AA where people can go to 'dry out'.

Which really has the country confused about 'doing it'. In fact, the once-sacrosanct institution of marriage is now under intense scrutiny. 'Honest couples prepared to talk about intimacy' are being hounded down by magazines and TV networks to discuss what goes on in the so-called nuptial bed.

This goes hand in hand with another trend which is burgeoning across America and parts of Europe: home-made sex movies – as in watching your neighbours at it. Recently, an industry has sprung up which provides erotic home-movies to couples who want to watch what other couples literally get up to behind closed doors. It's certainly one way of having those nagging questions answered.

As the country grapples with the question: How Much? How Often? I would like to quote from a religious book that has been in my family for generations which gives the biblical answer to what should and shouldn't go on in a marriage regarding sex.

The book, which interprets laws of the Old Testament, says the following:

'It is written (Exodus 21:10) *And her conjugal rights, shall he not diminish.*

'Men of a strong constitution who enjoy the pleasures of life, having profitable pursuits at home and are tax exempt, should perform their marital duty nightly. Labourers who work in the town where they reside, should perform their marital duty twice weekly; but if they are employed in another town, only once a week. Merchants who travel into villages with their mules, to buy grain to be sold in town, and others like them, should perform their marital duty once a week. Men who convey freight on camels from distant places, should attend to their marital duty once in thirty days.'

I believe this will go a long way to providing the answers the inquisitive mind is looking for.

G SPOT

Poor men. They really thought they were making progress in the complex and dangerous world that is female sexuality.

Like lemmings to the sea they have spent the past couple of years throwing themselves enthusiastically at the G spot. With courage and torch in hand they have gone off exploring treacherous terrain. Many have been seriously maimed in the process, falling from a towering bed and cracking the skull, or being smashed in the face by a thrashing knee.

Many have been disillusioned and defeated, unable to hold their heads up in public due to feelings of failure. Still, mankind has pressed on in search of that elusive pot of gold, that mysterious Eden that so many have sought and so few found.

Many G spot explorers have ended up around my coffee table, feeling forlorn, grossly inadequate and shell-shocked in this New Age era of pleasing women. They begged me for maps to help them navigate the unpredictable peaks and troughs while their women-folk grew impatient. 'Hoy! How much longer you gonna be? Go left. Left, you fool, not right.'

Then a strange and wonderful thing started happening. 'Eureka!' men started yelling at me over the phone. 'I found it!' Someone had cracked the code and spread the good news around: 'It's to the right of centre!'

But men's joy was short lived. Just when G spots were being uncovered in yuppie households all around Australia, a new movie was being released which would reduce men's gallant efforts to nought. Now women have a new and more complex set of demands.

Sacred Sex is a documentary about the newest sex sensation. The latest word out of the US is that sex should no longer be genital based. Annie Sprinkle, sex goddess and one of the stars of the film, describes it thus: 'Sex is almost exactly like food. There is junk sex, health sex and gourmet sex.'

Genital sex is junk sex. Bye bye G spot. Sacred sex is the higher form of 'gourmet' sex. It is spiritual according to its practitioners. It brings people closer to God. It is modelled on ancient sex rituals as outlined in the Karma Sutra and other mystic, secret, Eastern texts. Most importantly, it feels fantastic.

It is more a meditation than an act. A couple, by using breathing and meditation techniques, takes the rising sexual energy and directs it up the base of their spines towards the brain. The energy travels up through various energy points inside the body called 'chakras'. When it finally hits the brain, the mind explodes in ecstasy.

This explosion is akin to an orgasm only it's in the head not between the legs and can last one to two hours. In the film, one woman is seen to be having a mind-blowing mind-'gasm or *full-body orgasm*. The only connection between herself and lover is his foot which is placed on her chest, otherwise known as the 'heart chakra'. He is channelling his energy into her chakra and it most certainly seems to be working.

So suddenly every woman I know wants one. Has to have one. Is grabbing their men's legs as they walk in the front door and trying to milk the left foot for every last drop of energy. Being New Age and ever-vigilant in the area of satisfying women's needs, men desperately want to oblige.

My husband, feeling fabulous and mighty heroic from having discovered my G spot, is ready and willing to explore the next uncharted terrain. He says he's going to give me the newest, hottest, hippest 'gasm in town. I warn him in advance: 'You are not allowed to touch me sexually, okay? You have to try and unlock my erotic energy at the base of my spine and bring it up through my chakras, okay?'

'Sure, babe,' he says, enthusiastically, not knowing what the hell I am talking about. Men never do know what we want, and they never admit that they don't. He sits, staring into my eyes, with his leg stupidly on my chest wondering where this new chakra spot is supposed to be.

'Concentrate. Focus your energy,' I whisper, leaning back and breathing rapidly like the woman in the movie. 'Unleash my erotic potential. Open my heart chakra! Open my chakra!' I yell.

Unfortunately, he gets totally baffled. He forgets that we are talking about gourmet sex not junk sex and does a very junky thing. He grabs my nipple with his foot and squeezes it passionately between his toes in a bid to turn me on.

'Ahhhh!' I scream jumping out of my skin, brutally transmogrified from my spiritual meditation back into a state of junkiness.

'I told you not to touch me sexually!' I sob. 'And take your hands away from my Yoni! This is not about junk, genital sex! It's spiritual. You've ruined my Karma,' I say storming off to sulk.

So now men are sitting around my coffee tables begging for maps of the new 'chakra spot' or the 'C' spot as one poor guy dubbed it. But I should warn them.

Having now done a couple of sacred sex workshops, I have discovered how to drive the energy up the spine and have a 'mind-'gasm'. I can honestly say this: It's safe, it's clean, it feels unbelievably wonderful, and best of all you can do it on your own. As in no man need apply. Unless guys want to render themselves redundant, I suggest they stop trying so hard to help us women discover our sacred sexuality.

LOVE STRUCK

'There is more than one kind of love', say the words of a well-known rock song.

So who am I to scorn at the sounds of love pouring from the mouths of marauding hordes outside my window. The burbled hiccups, the yells of 'f…ing beauties', as drunken rabble spill into my street (next to the Hawthorn football club) in Melbourne the night of the Grand Final.

They are in love. Not my kind of love, but love none the less. Love bordering on worship. The muffled cries and squeals from pissed fans as touching in their own way as the sounds a mother makes on seeing her child walk, a lover on receiving the long awaited proposal.

'Ya f…ing c…ts' rings out over the crowd as one fan affectionately praises his winning team in his own personal and very special dialogue of love.

'F…ing bloody Hawks. Good on yers,' yells another of the

yellow and brown tribe of creatures passing under my window with balloons, scarves, hats and all other manner of baggage hanging off them, talking in strange tongues: 'Awww... yeahhh.'

There are now about ten thousand people in my street. Ten thousand love-struck people bumping into poles, smashing their cars into other cars in a bid to try to pass each other by in the narrow lane. All sense of reason and perspective gone. Watching them reminds me of the sort of romantic infatuations I had as a teenager. Their adoration is almost mystical.

Horns are honking, bottles are smashing. Particularly noteworthy are horns that play tunes. Like some deranged opera there are ten different tunes going at once as car loads of revellers seek to assert their individuality. To be something for a night.

The sound of glass under tyre rings in the air. I watch a man vomit on the pavement outside my window. Another pisses against the lamp post. Then I watch a group of kids across the road trying to pull a spike out of the neighbour's wooden fence. It is a reminder of what love does to the human spirit. Liberation is in the air. A celebration of life. A time for Mr and Mrs Australia and the kids to break out of the harness of 'ideal citizen' – just this once, in the ensuing exhilaration.

A small group starts bashing at a neighbour's fence. 'Tear down the picket fence. Come out of your houses and unite', is the catch-cry. This is middle-Australia's Berlin Wall.

I have been prepared all day to be in deep hate. In hate, hate, hate with the noisy, beer-swilling, traffic-making fans who would keep me up for two days. I cursed and awaited mass destruction. Bolting the doors, switching on the alarm and waiting to be highly annoyed.

It is not the case. I'm deeply touched as the lovesick herd

begin singing some mottled, maudlin version of what sounds like the Hawthorn theme song: 'We are the mighty fighting Hawks...(burble, warble)...'

I begin burbling out the Hawthorn song too, even though I dislike football. I swanker merrily around my living room even though I am not drunk. 'Awwwww ya f...g shit,' someone screams piercing the night air as another glass shatters. I hope it is not the stained glass window. Love is often like this. After the exhilaration comes the let-down. The '*Is that all there is?*' of Peggy Lee. And then the anger, as the disappointment returns.

Those happy, love-struck people in my street are going to have to come down. On Monday they are all returning to work or to unemployment, or to their mediocre marriages and scouring bosses. They will have to face the unhappy reality that their *objet d'amour*, their treasured beloved, is not going to save them from themselves or from their own tired lives. That the moments of passion in life are but fleeting, ephemeral gifts.

A punch, a bash, a shattered window, alleviates the anger before a train ride back to the outer suburbs of disillusionment.

I decide to go off to Mother's, the other side of town. It is safer to leave before things get messy. Police vans have already started to parade up and down. Impending violence is in the air. I have never liked sticking about for the morning after passion, preferring to grab my things and split before the harsh light of day hits. Split whilst I still feel hot and sweaty and flushed with excitement of love.

As I get into my car I fear for the fans in my street. I fear for their romantic souls. For I know that like me, they will grown far, far too sober as the hours of their lives tick on.

LETTERS

Dear Ruth,

I am a single male, average height, build, and aged in my forties. I am also bisexual. In my view, the best way to spruce up your sex-life is to be kinky, like me. I wear Latex rubber gloves. Latex fits like a second skin, and the smell is better than perfume.

P.K., GLENORCHY, TAS

Dear Ruth,

What a relief to actually read in a mainstream newspaper that I am not so strange after all. I have enjoyed rubber clothing for as long as I can remember. Even as a child. I am glad people are becoming more accepting of differences. One day I may even be able to tell my wife. We have been married for twenty-two years and apart from my rubber interest, our sex-life is normal.

RON C., (FRUIT MARKETS), THORNLEIGH, NSW

Ruth,

In your piece on fantasies, you omitted mentioning the one that I've been most asked about – the ever-popular 'threesome' of two women and a man. I've been working in the sex industry for seven years, and yes, I've encountered clients who have the foot fetish or 'let's pretend we're on a tropical island and you're a native virgin girl'. But it is the threesome that has kept a lot of us in business.

C.H., PADDINGTON, NSW

Dear Ruth,

Your article on turn-ons reminded me of a woman I dated. She had a small silk blanket that she would place on the pillow before we made love. She would rub her face on the blanket whilst I did my duty from behind. Maybe this wasn't as silly as it sounds, as she always had incredible orgasms.

BRAD, ESSENDON, WA

Dear Ruth,

My wife and I have been married for forty years. We have always had good sex, as my wife decided from day one that she was going to be the domineering one. What I mean by this is that she administered the strap to my bare bottom before we had intercourse. Doing this seems to make her hot for sex, and our lovemaking is still as hot as it was on our wedding night.

MR G., RICHMOND, NSW

Dear Ruth,

I would like to see my wife making love to another woman. Initially she was taken aback, but has since mellowed to the idea although finding someone to go along with the idea is another problem. I'm hoping this fantasy will eventuate although I can understand if it does not, and I was wondering if any of your readers have had similar ideas.

PETER T., CAMPBELLTOWN, NSW

Dear Ruth,

I read your articles and letters with interest. One letter really astounded me. Every man *can* totally satisfy his woman by using his mouth and his tongue. As long as he does it slowly and softly, never fast and keeps on doing this until she has had an orgasm. The copulation afterwards can only be a success. I hope the doctor who wrote to you will find out about this, to help those desperate men.

MRS N., ADELAIDE, SA

Dear Ruth,

I have never understood how anyone in their right mind, could engage in oral sex. When Mrs N. described it last week in your column, I wondered if she would be just as willing to clean the inside of her toilet bowl with her tongue.

JOHN C. W., STRATHPINE, QLD

Madam,

So John M. loves oral sex – all versions – and sees his wife's genitals as one of his favourite places. Good luck to him for having such a cooperative partner, but has he considered the risks and what hidden dangers lurk when the recreation park is so close to the sewage outfall?

K.T., HYDE PARK, QLD

Dear Ruth,

I am twenty-eight years old and partake in 'self-pleasure' quite regularly and absolutely love it! I like to wear my stiletto heels as they make me feel very sexy and I seem to get a much deeper lasting orgasm whilst I wear them. Do any other women have similar fantasies? I hope I'm not alone in enjoying these pleasures.

L.D., DARWIN, NT

Dear Ruth,

A Pleasure Positive Party? You've got my vote. We all need to spend more time pleasuring ourselves. It's free, it's fun and it feels wonderful. If this makes me guilty, I can only say I will be a repeat offender.

SUE, GOSFORD, NSW

Dear Ruth Ostrow,

I use prostitutes on a regular basis. I had an unsuccessful marriage, and have tried personal adds without success. Since I am afraid of intimacy I get more satisfaction out of having a prostitute beat me with a cane or whip than having sex. I have found prostitutes more helpful and understanding than most psychiatrists.

'P', SYDNEY, NSW

Dear Ruth,

I am a 'screamer' whilst making love, and I can tell you that my partner gets very aroused hearing me scream in ecstasy.

J.J., CASUARINA, NT

Dear Ruth,

To all those who married screamers. Half your luck. I married the sack of potatoes who shut the garden gate twenty-five years ago.

EX-SPUD DIGGER, SA

Madam,

To those screaming alley cat females who like everyone to know they are indulging in sexual intercourse. I suggest a good cold bucket of water thrown over them would jolt them back into behaving like decent, civilised human beings.

ARTHUR, CABOOLTURE, QLD

Dear Ruth,

There seems to be a lot of women out there who are having trouble achieving orgasm. May I suggest they try anal sex with their partner. I was a little bit sceptical when my boyfriend first suggested it to me, but now I'm a total convert – it's fantastic! I strongly recommend it to women of all ages.

KYLIE, SA

Dear Ruth,

I read your article about fantasies and would like to share an experience I had with an ex-girlfriend of mine. We discovered by accident that we both had a fixation with doctors. After much discussion we realised we had been in hospital as children – I for my tonsils, she for a toe operation. After much laughter we decided to act on our fantasies. Yes, it's true. We played doctors and nurses and it was a real turn-on.

A.N., BONDI, NSW

The Editor,

I would like to complain about the disgusting explicit sex articles in Ruth Ostrow's column. She should not be allowed to write them. She is talking about people making noises during sex. We should be talking about love and loyalty.

A.E., WELLINGTON, NSW

Dear Ruth,

Masturbation is a mortal sin. To set out to satisfy your body by yourself is completely evil.

M.S., MOONEE PONDS, VIC

Dear Ruth,

In response to your writer from Moonee Ponds, VIC. If masturbation is a mortal sin, why didn't God put our genitals between our shoulder blades, instead of between our legs?

ANON., TOOWOOMBA, QLD

Dear Ruth,

Spare a thought for me as a sexually active male with a medical disorder that I have to live with which makes me reliant on having to wear nappies. Self-masturbation is my only pleasure as women are not turned on when confronted with a thirty-five-year-old wearing a nappy and plastic pilchers. I would love to be embraced and have the pleasure of making love to an understanding lady. I have never paid for sex and never will, as I feel it would make my handicap feel worse than what it already is.

JOHN, GOLD COAST, QLD

Dear Ruth,

I would like to know why is pornography such a bad thing when it helps me learn about sex and how to enjoy it to the fullest? I am a twenty-nine-year-old mother of three and the role of sex with my husband was just a quick job and it was all over and done with. But now I have a new partner and I am experiencing sex in many different and erotic ways. Why is all this locked in the closet?

SUSY, CENTRAL QLD

Dear Ruth,

I am writing to you about anal sex as your paper never mentions anything about it. Having sex in the back hole is beautiful. I am married for ten years now and my wife and I have been doing anal sex very regularly in those years as well as normal sex. We both love it! Some people might think it wouldn't be nice, but I bet there's quite a lot of couples doing it. But no-one says anything about it.

JOHN, MILDURA, VIC

Hello Ruth,

Last Thursday evening on the TV a rather nice lady on the *Sex* program was going on about various places on the body to fondle, kiss and lick. Anyway, it set me off with the giggles and when she mentioned the 'rim of the anus', I exploded with laughter. I mean to say, young Ruth, this puts an entirely new meaning to the saying 'you can kiss my arse'. Should one's partner 'backfire' at that given moment, I guess one could land up on the top of the wardrobe.

GEORGE, BEDFORDALE, WA

Dear Ruth,

I am a man in my late twenties with strong desires to indulge in anal penetration. I do this with fruits and vegetables and dildos. I don't think that I'm homosexual, but I have occasionally allowed gays to penetrate me because it feels terrific. My only problem is the looseness of the sphincter. But do you think that it is normal for a guy to enjoy this activity?

ANON., SYDNEY, NSW